Instructor's
Resource Manual for

EFFECTIVE
MANAGEMENT
IN NURSING

THIRD EDITION

JoAnne Alexander
Mary Kay Hermann
Christine Schutz
Sheila Trimble
Phillip J. Decker
Eleanor J. Sullivan

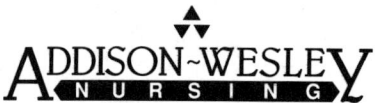

A Division of the Benjamin/Cummings Publishing Company, Inc.
Redwood City, California • Menlo Park, California
Reading, Massachusetts • New York • Don Mills, Ontario • Wokingham, U.K.
Amsterdam • Bonn • Sydney • Singapore • Tokyo • Madrid • San Juan

Project Editor: Bradley Burch

Production Coordinator: Eleanor Renner Brown

Project Support: Patricia Walters, Kathleen Sloan, Sandra M. Handley

ISBN   0-8053-7864-2
 2345678910-BK-95949392

Addison-Wesley Nursing
A Division of the Benjamin/Cummings Publishing Company, Inc.
390 Bridge Parkway
Redwood City, CA   94065

TABLE OF CONTENTS

Introduction to the Texts

This Instructor's Manual and the Student Workbook contain a compendium of action-oriented learning activities in which students practice using ideas and strategies covered in dept in the text. Through individual and small group exercises, inventories, simulations, assessment tools, and questionnaires, the theory-practice connection is promoted. Students actually live through, or experience, the interpersonal phenomena about which they have read. Learning is enhanced through this experiential mode. In addition to learning theory and practice specific to nursing management, students will learn about values, how they influence nursing care, and how personal attributes influence the role of each manager.

Instructors can use this manual as an adjunct to lectures and discussions and as an integral part of experiences off campus and on campus. While the workbook has been prepared as a companion to the text, it can readily be used along or with an alternative text with minimal sequencing.

LEVEL OF THE STUDENT WORKBOOK

Student workbooks and instructor's guides are generally directed to the needs of a single level of students. This one, on the contrary, is geared to all levels of students--in diploma, associate degree, baccalaureate, RN second-step, and graduate programs--and to practitioners of nursing as well. The tools and activities are appropriate to both undergraduate and graduate nursing curricula, depending on the depth and breadth of responses expected of the students. They may also be used selectively in in-service education programs for nursing managers and potential managers.

USING THE TEXTBOOK TO FULL ADVANTAGE

This manual is one element of a three-part set. The three components--workbook, instructor's manual, and text--form a complete package for teaching nursing management, either as a separate course or as an integrated thread in a nursing curriculum.

The text is a contemporary and comprehensive approach to the content and concepts of nursing management, emphasizing a holistic approach. The instructor's manual, keyed to the text chapter by chapter, offers the instructor all the customary materials required in nursing course syllabi, including topical lecture outlines, higher order questions for seminar and conference discussion, and references to the complementary learning activities in the workbook.

Each exercise, inventory, simulation, assessment tool, and questionnaire in the workbook is thoroughly explained, to minimize the coordination tasks of the instructor. An instructor with a large group of students can thus have them work in several small groups independently for heightened learning and discussion. Students and faculty can easily locate all the materials that each structured

1

learning activity requires. Theoretical background for each tool is available in the text.

It is recommended that instructors review each learning activity before assigning it to determine how to use it most effectively. Some are designed as intrapersonal exercises, which the individual student may choose to share with the instructor or with peers. It is suggested that the choice to share be left to the student, to allow for personal privacy and to encourage greater honesty in answering questions. Other tools may be used in dyads, triads, or small groups. The instructor may wish to bring all students together for a discussion period as well. Guidelines for discussion have been provided for appropriate tools.

Some of the exercises and inventories may produce anxiety or be stressful for students. In those cases, supportive action by the instructor may be helpful.

All of the exercises can be used in a shorter form; that is, portions can be deleted to produce half-hour or shorter exercises. This is especially true with the role plays.

How to Use This Manual

The Instructor's Manual is designed to supplement Effective Management in Nursing, 3rd Edition and Nursing Management: An Experiential/Skill-Building Workbook. The latter contains 45 experiential exercises and can be used in training and certificate programs for nurse managers/supervisors or in baccalaureate or master's nursing programs. The experiential exercises consist of roleplays, self-assessments, group discussions and small group experiences.

This manual also contains several items that will help to plan classroom assignments, provide conceptual background to participants, and manage the learning environment in order to increase participant learning. In the experiential learning method, the instructor/trainer is not so much a transmitter of knowledge; rather, the instructor serves as a resource person, coach, and facilitator.

The classroom that uses this approach will be noisier and less structured than the one using traditional methods of lecture. The experiential method allows participants the opportunity for more self-awareness and active involvement in learning. A structure is provided for each exercise; however, the instructor must resist the temptation to provide too much rigid adherence to is because this may defeat the purpose of learning by self-discovery.

Additionally, this manual contains a number of other items that are helpful to instructors using the experiential method. Helpful hints for facilitating group experiences are included as well as clear descriptions of the methods used throughout the book, i.e., self-assessments, roleplays, small groups, and discussions. A test bank and transparency masters are also provided.

2

Teaching Methods

FACILITATING GROUP EXPERIENCE

Experiential learning is quite different from the traditional classroom lecture method. The following is a list of the major aspects of experiential learning.

1. The primary focus of responsibility for learning is shifted from the instructor to the participant.

2. More than cognitive processes are involved, i.e., participants become involved behaviorally and affectively as well.

3. The goals for learning involve developing skills and attitudes as well as the goal of imparting knowledge.

4. The participant is active both physically and psychologically.

Because of the differences between the traditional and experiential methods, there is a special set of "do's" and "don'ts" for the instructor using the exercises in this manual.

1. Remember that the instructor sets the tone of the class experience to a great degree. You are a role model and should facilitate serious participation by participants.

2. Be sure that participants understand the procedure and the theoretical issues before beginning. Allow them to ask questions first.

3. Remain flexible. Much of what occurs in experiential learning is spontaneous and individualized. Therefore, there will be less order and structure in the classroom.

4. Allow for moderate physical movement and noise, which indicate a comfortable and good learning environment.

5. Read over the directions and know what is to be expected. This avoids chaos in the classroom and allows you to do some planning in spite of the spontaneity involved in each exercise.

6. Keep notes on reactions to and effectiveness of the exercise. This allows you to tailor the exercises to your needs, to correct problems that may occur, and to record what went well so that it can be repeated.

7. Don't hesitate to use the exercises that fit for you or parts of exercises that you think will best meet your course objectives.

Understanding the use of groups is essential to experiential learning in the classroom. Using small groups allows for more social contact and affiliation and enables participants to learn from each other. In general, the instructor should observe the following things in the various classroom groups:

1. Whether participants are prepared for group discussions/activities.

2. Whether participants know the group goals.

3. Whether participants adhere to basic communication rules such as one person speaking at a time, using "I statements," and listening to each other.

4. Which participants seem uninvolved or silently angry or do most of the talking.

5. Which participants prefer more leadership functions.

The tasks of the instructor are to assist participants in meeting their goals, involve them all as much as possible and be sure that they are prepared for the exercises. For many of the exercises, preparation prior to class will be necessary in order to complete them properly.

The Use of Classroom Physical Space

For the exercises in this manual, no unusual classroom equipment or layout is required. However, the following things are helpful for most exercises:

1. A room large enough to hold all participants.

2. Moveable chairs for doing triad work or small group work.

3. Blackboards or other writing space that is visible to all.

4. Each participant comes to class without paper, pencil and his/her student workbook.

Small group meeting rooms can be helpful, but are not necessary. An alternative waiting area for participants outside the classroom is necessary for some exercises. Special equipment or materials beyond the above are described for each exercise.

Implementing Exercises in Large Classes

There are some advantages to small class sizes when using these exercises. For example, there is greater involvement and greater participant-to-participant interaction, more individualized instruction, and greater likelihood of discussion. Nevertheless, these exercises can be adopted to large classes either by the use of small group work or modifying the triad role-play method. For most exercises, the triad role-play method is suggested; however, for larger classes, a presentation of a roleplay by the instructor to the entire class may be more feasible.

To facilitate small group work in a large class, the instructor can have each group designate a spokesperson who summarizes the small group's actions to the whole group. Discussion questions after the exercise can center around differences between groups.

Competition among small groups can add to the involvement and meaningfulness of an exercise. Also, when there are many groups, different parts of the exercises can be assigned to different groups in order to save time. Larger classes may need more group processing time; however, few of the exercises will require more work beyond the classroom for the instructor because of the larger size of a class.

METHODS USED IN THE EXERCISES

1.   Self-Assessments

There are several exercises that utilize questionnaires or other self-assessment devices which have many advantages in teaching nursing management. First, self-assessments are simple ways to teach theory and concepts. Participants are asked to respond to questions that measure their attitudes or behaviors which are relevant to concepts in nursing management. This allows for involvement and interest in theory as it personally applies to each person.

Additionally, self-assessments give useful information to the student about him/herself that can be integrated into other aspects of his/her self-image. These devices allow a person to be distinguished from others and to be compared with established norms.

Some instructors may have experienced negative responses to using self-assessment devices. If these are anticipated, they can be considerably reduced. One problem is that participants may fear that their results will become known to others. This is an understandable concern for privacy that can be honored by encouraging participants to share their scores in small groups and with people they feel they can trust. Sometimes participants won't want to share their results. This refusal should be accepted by the instructor. Nevertheless, if the instructor self-discloses, it will be easier for participants to share with each other.

Another issue which can cloud the use of self-assessments is that participants may think that the devices don't measure anything of "real meaning." This can be curtailed by showing how the instruments are related to human behavior and nursing management on a practical level by giving real world examples to which the class members can relate. Also, it is necessary for the instructor to be prepared to explore reasons why test results may not fit for a person, e.g., rating errors, misunderstood directions, changes in reliability and validity of responses across situations.

5

Finally, the devices used in this training manual do not emphasize social desirability, but individuals ma interpret them in that manner. To avoid this, tell participants that there is no right or wrong set of responses and that there should be differences among individuals. Encourage people to feel "okay" about their personal responses.

2. Role Plays

The advantages for using role playing as a learning device are numerous and have been well established in research. Role playing helps a participant to examine another person's point of view. Additionally, role playing allows for the introduction of a problem or situation for discussion or study. Ineffective behaviors, attitudes, or values of the participants can be pointed out. In triad role plays, this is accomplished through the observer role. The observer's task is to follow the guidelines for the role play and to give constructive, specific feedback to the others in the triad. If the class has not used role plays previously, a discussion on how to give feedback is in order. Describing the person's actions and comparing them to the guidelines or key behaviors is emphasized. Critical, judgmental or sarcastic feedback is not appropriate.

In role plays, participants are highly involved in the experience of learning. Role playing engages the learner in a dramatic way and stimulates thinking and feeling. Participants can gain insight without dealing with the possible harmful effects of real life situations. Role playing is a safe way to try out new behaviors and new solutions.

In this manual, all role plays have guidelines/key behaviors to assist participants in their experience. Also, brief situations or scenarios are often provided that are taken from realistic events in nursing management. Participants may choose their own scenes to role play, but be sure they choose relevant, appropriate situations.

Role plays can also be done as a class demonstration. The instructor can choose class members to assist in a role play in front of the class. The rest of the class can be "observers" and provide feedback. This method allows the instructor more control over the learning experience, but creates less involvement on the part of each individual. A class demonstration role play can be used instead of, or in addition to, triad role plays. If class demonstration is used, be sure the players clearly understand their roles, put a time limit on the sequence, and allow the class plenty of time to discuss the sequence thoroughly.

Another alternative to triad role plays is an expansion of the class demonstration role play to include as many other participants as time allows, i.e., more than one role play takes place before the entire class. After each role play, the class provides feedback to the players. The players select one of the observers' ideas for improving the role play and they reenact the situation. This method allows each of the players to practice a new improved version of the role plays, but reduces the involvement of other participants compared to the triad method.

In general, the triad method provides for the most participant involvement of the methods discussed here, but the least control by the instructor. Although the instructor monitors by walking around the class and watching the various triad groups, in a larger class, it is difficult to get to all groups. For this reason, triad role plays are not recommended with other 35 members. A class demonstration role play or the expanded version of this is more likely to be successful. One disadvantage to using role plays is that some participants may be too shy or self-centered to profit from them. Learning may be hard to evaluate and individually determined; also, much time is utilized. Nevertheless, careful monitoring and the use of key behaviors can curtail some of these problems. Role playing is always, however, time consuming, which is to be expected for any experiential learning to take place.

3.   Behavior Modeling Training

Often behavior modeling is used instead of role playing. Behavior modeling training consists of the procedures outlines in social learning theory: imitation of effective behaviors; use of retention aids; intensive and guided practice of new and unfamiliar behavior; reinforcement or recognition for application of the specific behaviors; and transfer of training principles.

In the first step of behavior modeling training, the instructor presents a videotape or film, called a modeling display, to the trainees. The modeling display shows two persons interacting, usually a supervisor and a subordinate. The supervisor, or model, is demonstrating the key behavior, a learning point, to be taught to the trainees. The modeling performance should concisely and distinctly demonstrate the desirable behavior in handling a specific job situation. Most important in the modeling performance, the model must be reinforced for performing the model behaviors.

The second step of behavior modeling training involves retention aids. Retention aids include (a) the trainees' reading descriptions of the key behaviors to be presented in the modeling display; (b) the trainees' viewing the modeling display demonstrating the key behaviors; and (c) the trainees' mentally rehearsing the key behaviors they have read and seen, picturing themselves performing them with one of their own employees.

The third step of behavior modeling training is behavior rehearsal, or supervised reenactment of the model performance. At this step, trainees practice skills they have seen modeled until they are proficient at these skills.

Trainees are divided into groups of three or four in order to simulate a real work situation as nearly as possible, provide as nonthreatening an environment as possible, and enable each trainee to role-play as often as possible.

The fourth step of behavior modeling training is reinforcement. Trainers orally reinforce trainees' appropriate behavior as often and as clearly as possible immediately following behavior performance. Observers orally reinforce trainees' solutions to problems and support trainers' feedback on key behaviors. Trainees pride themselves when their behavior favorably imitates behavior on the modeling display. Trainees also see other trainees praised for proper behavior. Finally, trainees often praise each other.

The fifth and final step in behavior modeling training involves transfer principles, so that learning can be transferred from behavior rehearsal to actual job performance. Transfer is accomplished through self-reinforcement or social reinforcement on the job. In self-reinforcement, the trainees themselves recognize their success in transferring the model's behavior to their own behavior in an actual work situation. In social reinforcement, the trainees' supervisor recognizes their appropriate performance and clearly indicates that recognition to the trainees.

For more information on behavioral modeling, see Decker, P.J. & Nathan, B., (1985), <u>Behavior Modeling Training: Principles and Applications</u>. New York: Praeger.

4. <u>Large Group Discussion</u>

Both small and large group discussions allow for the presentation of views, opinions or expertise on the part of participants as well as the instructor. The instructor can also use discussions to help change attitudes by persuasion and examination of information or to explore solutions to problems.

Some advantages are that discussions allow for the pooling of the knowledge and abilities of many people, two-way communication, and feedback between the class and the instructor. The following are guidelines for leading a large group discussion:

1. Make a brief statement about the purpose of the discussion.

2. Play the "devil's advocate" and respectfully challenge participant's statements.

3. Encourage participation by all participants, e.g., ask quieter people to comment on a previous remark or summarize the discussion.

4. Redirect the discussion to keep participants on the subject.

5. Keep alert to verbal and nonverbal cues of the group members.

As a discussion leader, the instructor should be more controlling and directing than when monitoring triads or facilitating small group experiences.

5.   ## Small Group Experience

In small group activities, participants interact more with each other; the instructor's role is to make sure that the group is able to perform as efficiently as possible. The instructor must be sure all directions are understood clearly before the activity begins. When individuals ask questions, give answers carefully in order to avoid telling people too much. Try to avoid jumping in on small group experiences. It is better to let participants learn for themselves. Observing the groups and pointing out problems in group processes should be done carefully. People may become defensive and not respond well to your comments. However, you can use what you see to indirectly stimulate discussion in the small groups or in the group as a whole. Finally, the instructor should provide plenty of positive reinforcement and reassurance to group members.

Use of Student Workbook in Courses

The student workbook (Nursing Management: An Experiential/Skill-Building Workbook) can be used for instruction in a management course offered for credit in a college or university nursing program, in a continuing education noncredit course, or in a hospital noncredit course leading to a management certificate. Below is a description and schedule for use of this text in (1) a credit course and (2) a noncredit program.

Credit Course:

The workbook is an excellent tool for instruction in most nursing educational programs. It is particularly useful in a generic baccalaureate program or a Bachelor of Science in Nursing program designed for registered nurses. It may also be used in an associate degree or diploma program if management skill development is a component of the curriculum. For graduate students whose career goals include management, this book would also be appropriate.

The major strength of the workbook is that it teaches the student actual management skills in a number of realistic situations. The student practices the skill and receives feedback on his/her performance in a controlled, simulated setting. This is not unlike the manner in which nursing students learn other skills. This augments the student's learning in the classroom and enables him/her to put into practice the skills discussed in class.

Additionally, the workbook is based on known principles appropriate for teaching the adult learner. These include the ability to (1) determine one's own readiness to learn; (2) integrate new learning in a base of experience; (3) be self-directing; and (4) apply new knowledge in the immediate future.

9

The following is a typical schedule for integration of laboratory learning activities (using the workbook) into a three-credit hour course in nursing management. The class meets once a week for three hours.

Class Schedule

Week	Activity	Location
1	Orientation	Classroom
2-4	Lecture and discussion	Classroom
5-9	Skill development	Laboratory
10-14	Clinical experience	Hospital
15	Clinical conference summary	Classroom
16	Final Exam	Classroom

There are, of course, many variations of this schedule that could be used. This one offers a concentration of activities, lecture, or laboratory and does the following: (1) course content is presented first; (2) practice of the skills appropriate to the theoretical content is presented in the laboratory next; (3) practice takes place in a clinical setting with a nurse manager (usually head nurse) utilized as the student's preceptor; and (4) integration of content with skill development and practice is reviewed in a final summary conference.

The exercises could also be spaced out in such a course, especially if taught 2 days a week. Lecture could be done the first day and an exercise the second. Either way, it is suggested that one exercise per section be used.

Noncredit Use

Many hospitals may wish to use the workbook to structure a nurse supervisor "certificate" course in which trainees are given a certificate for covering 80-90% of the modules offered in a long program.

Such a supervisory certificate training program is usually designed for employees who have recently been promoted to supervisor as well as for seasoned supervisors who desire to upgrade their skills in the latest techniques and principles of supervision and management.

A certificate training program consists of 10 to 15 three-hour classes, a total of 30 to 45 hours of instruction. Each class covers a selected topic critical to the role of the supervisor. The entire program should focus on two major areas: (1) basic supervisory skills and (2) interpersonal skills.

Each student who successfully completes the entire program within a period of one year should receive a certificate.

A certificate training program is designed to be flexible, and to fit conveniently in the busy schedules of supervisors. A 3-hour morning section from 9:00 a.m. to noon is possible.

The entire program takes 13 to 15 weeks to complete, meeting an average of once a week. The total program is offered once a year, allowing supervisors to make up classes that are missed, thereby meeting the certification requirements.

Such a certificate program would include the following sections that would incorporate approximately one hour of lecture (from our text), one-and-a-half hours of exercises from the workbook, and a half hour of breaks and question answering:

1. Organizational theory
2. Roles and self-esteem
3. Communication
4. Assertiveness
5. Leadership
6. Decision making and problem solving
7. Motivation
8. Time management and stress
9. Employment Selection
10. Staff development
11. Employee appraisal
12. Labor relations
13. Survival skills

Optional:

14. Dealing with higher management
15. Emerging issues

You will notice that these modules conform to the sections of the workbook. Such a course can be extremely useful for teaching management skills to nurse managers.

S E C T I O N I

**CHAPTER OUTLINES
AND TOPICS FOR DISCUSSION**

CHAPTER 1

Introduction to Nursing Management

Chapter Outline

   I. Introduction

  II. Key Issues for Health Care in the 1990s
     A. Economics
     B. Competitive nature of the industry
     C. Shortages of health care professional personnel
     D. Focus on quality outcomes and consumerism

 III. Key Issues for Nursing Managers in the 1990s
     A. Need for effective leadership
     B. Development of standards
     C. Expertise in practice
     D. Empowerment
     E. Codependency
     F. Authority, responsibility, accountability
     G. Effective communication

Topics for Discussion

1. Define accountability as related to the goals of nursing. What methods does society have for maintaining the accountability of its members?

2. Discuss the role of the nurse manager as it relates to patient care.

3. Discuss the role of nurse manager as it relates to nursing research.

4. Compare productivity in nursing in the 1980s and 1990s.

5. Discuss the character of nursing units.

CHAPTER 2

The Nature of Organizations in Health Care

Chapter Outline

I. The Nature of Organizational Theory
   A. Complexity, formalization, centralization
   B. Katz & Kahn's open system theory
      1. Input
      2. Throughput
      3. Output
      4. Cyclic events
      5. Negative entropy
      6. Information input
      7. Steady state
      8. Differentiation
      9. Integration
      10. Equifinality

II. Theories of Organization
   A. Classical theory
      1. Taylor
      2. Gilbreth
      3. Fayol
      4. Weber
   B. Neoclassical theory
      1. Follett
      2. Hawthorne studies
      3. Barnard
   C. Technological theory
      1. Woodward
   D. Modern systems theory
      1. Katz & Kahn
      2. March & Simon

III. Departmentalization

IV. Contingency Theory
   A. Environment
   B. Technology
   C. Strategy
   D. Organization structure
   E. People
   F. Interdependence
      1. pooled
      2. sequential
      3. reciprocal

V. Organizational Structure
   A. Functional structure
   B. Self-contained unit structure
   C. Matrix structure

D. Structures unique to health care

VI. Types of Health Care Organizations
   A. Acute care instructions
   B. Long term care institutions
   C. Ambulatory care organizations
   D. Home health care agencies
   E. Temporary health care services

VII. The Department of Nursing
   A. Shared governance

VIII. Organizational Effectiveness in Health Care Today
   A. Adaptability
   B. Organizational purpose
   C. Ability to test reality
   D. Integration

Topics for Discussion

1. Identify the potential environmental constraints of the nursing department (e.g., supply of nurses). How would each of these constraints influence the nursing department as a whole? The nursing units/floors?

2. Identify the input-throughput-output process within the nursing department. How is the nursing department affected by other organizational departments? How does the nursing department affect other organizational functions?

3. Identify several types of health care organizations. How may their inputs and outputs differ?

4. Discuss the concepts of horizontal and vertical organizational structure. Identify the location of the nursing department within both of these organizational dimensions.

5. Discuss several theories of organization. Compare and contrast them.

CHAPTER 3

The Functions of a Nurse Manager in Health Care Settings

Chapter Outline
I. Management Functions
   A. Planning
      1. Setting objectives
         a. Product/service objectives
         b. Efficiency objectives
         c. Social objectives
         d. Human resource objectives
      2. Evaluating the present situation and predicting future events
         a. Evaluation of internal environment
         b. Evaluation of external environment
   B. Organizing
      1. Authority and power
         a. Allocation rights
         b. Evaluation rights
      2. Bureaucracies
   C. Controlling
      1. Socialization
         a. Stages in the socialization process
            1) anticipatory socialization
            2) presocialization
            3) recruitment
            4) institutional socialization
            5) rite of passage
         b. Role transformation
      2. Managerial surveillance
         a. Direct observation
         b. Indirect observation
      3. Principles of control
   D. Decision making
      1. Problem identification
      2. Criteria selection
      3. Search for alternatives
      4. Evaluation of alternatives
      5. Selection of an alternative

II. Management Functions For The First-level Manager
   A. Planning
      1. Contingency planning
   B. Organizing
      1. Qualified and informed personnel
      2. Equipment
      3. Scheduling staff
      4. Patient care
   C. Controlling
      1. Intervention

16

Topics for Discussion

1. What is the importance of setting objectives? How would the absence of objectives in each of the four general areas (e.g., product/service) influence the nursing department? Present and discuss examples of objectives specific to nursing.

2. Describe the process of socialization. Using an example relevant to nursing, describe the movement through the five stages of this process. What are the implications for nursing management?

3. Discuss the relationship between the planning process and the establishment of organizational structure. Identify methods of organizing or coordinating (e.g., authority and power) and discuss the implications for nursing management (e.g., scheduling staff, training personnel).

CHAPTER 4

Organizing Care

Chapter Outline

    I. Introduction

   II. Delivery Systems
- A. Differentiated practice
- B. Case management
- C. Product line management
- D. Primary nursing
- E. Team nursing
- F. Functional nursing
- G. Total patient care

 III. Staffing and Scheduling
- A. Philosophy
- B. Productivity
- C. Accreditation requirements for staffing
- D. Flexible scheduling
- E. Supplemental staffing

  IV. Patient Classification
- A. Purposes
- B. GRASP
- C. MEDICOS
- D. Integration of care plan and classification system

Topics for Discussion

1. What is the importance of the nursing care delivery system? How does it affect nursing management?

2. What are the different delivery systems? Where are each found and why?

3. How do different systems of patient care delivery interact with hospital organization?

CHAPTER 5

Productivity

Chapter Outline

I. Introduction

II. What is Productivity
   A. Economic/industrial definitions
      1. Labor productivity statistic
      2. Total factor productivity measure
   B. Attempts to define productivity in health care
      1. The nature of health care inputs
      2. The nature of the institution's product
      3. Output or outcome

III. What is Nursing Productivity?
   A. Scientific management approach
   B. Systems framework approach

IV. Current Methods of Measuring Nursing Productivity
   A. Resources per patient day
      1. Standardizing patient days
   B. Degree of occupation
   C. Utilization rates
      1. Required hours of care as an input

V. Improving Nursing Productivity
   A. Changes in the use of inputs
      1. Matching supply with demand
      2. Making staff substitutions
      3. Controlling the use of supplies and equipment
   B. Changes in the care process
      1. Selected examples
      2. Documenting changes
      3. Calculating costs
      4. Measuring outcome
      5. Using the cost and outcome date

Topics for Discussion

1. Define productivity. Discuss methods of measuring it.

2. Discuss methods to improve nursing productivity.

CHAPTER 6

Ethics in Health Care

Chapter Outline

   I.   Prevalence of Ethical Issues

  II.   Ethics as Integral to Nursing Management
        A. Nurses obligations

 III.   Ethical Approaches
        A. Biomedical ethics
            1. Deontology
            2. Teleology

  IV.   Principles of Biomedical Ethics
        A. Autonomy
        B. Nonmaleficence
        C. Beneficence
        D. Justice

   V.   A Model for Addressing Ethical Issues
        A. Five steps
            1. Massage the dilemma
            2. Outline options
            3. Review criteria and resolve
            4. Affirm position and act
            5. Look back
        B. Application of the model to management
            decision making

  VI.   Special Issues for the Nurse Manager
        A. Providing safe care
        B. Confronting unsafe practice
        C. Supporting patient and staff autonomy
        D. Ethics education and resource management

Topics for Discussion

1. Why is ethics integral to nursing?

2. Discuss the different ethical approaches or philosophies.

3. Name and discuss the basic principles of biomedical ethics.

4. Discuss the 5-step model of ethics presented in the text.

5. Identify several special ethical issues for nurses and discuss each.

CHAPTER 7

Communication and Information Systems

Chapter Outline

    I. Introduction

   II. Theories of Communication

  III. Factors Influencing Management Communication
      A. Gender
      B. Societal culture
      C. Organizational culture

  IV. Effective Communication Through Human Interaction
      A. Principles of effective communication
      B. Oral communication
      C. Listening
      D. Written communication
      E. Distorted communication
      F. Assertiveness

   V. Special Types of Communication
      A. With subordinates
      B. With superiors
      C. With other health care personnel
      D. In public relations

  VI. Information Systems
      A. Patient monitoring
      B. Provision of care
      C. Patients records: charts, care plans and kardexes
      D. Training and evaluation
      E. Scheduling and staffing
      F. Communication with pharmacy, laboratory and radiology

  VII. Nursing Information Systems

 VIII. Hospital Information Systems

  IX. Nonhospital Systems

   X. Surviving with Computers

Topics for Discussion

1.   Discuss the importance of attending to both verbal and nonverbal communication. Discuss the potential problems resulting from incongruence between verbal and nonverbal communication.

2. What is active listing? Why is it important? What are the principles of active listening? Critique your listening skills.

3. Describe assertive behavior. What are the rules for assertive behavior? Using these rules as a guide, describe an example of assertive nurse manager behavior.

4. Identify the potential "receivers" of communication from the nurse manager "sender." In what direction does this communication flow (e.g., horizontal)? What strategies should the nurse manager use with each of these different "receivers"?

5. Identify situations in nursing in which group communication takes place. How may group members behave so that communication is facilitated? What behaviors of the group leader facilitate group communication?

6. Review the components of computers. Discuss the difference between hardware and software and the uses of each.

7. Discuss the various uses of computers within the total health care organization. How may the use of computers aid in patient care? How may these uses affect the nursing department?

8. Discuss the specific uses of computers within the nursing department (e.g., patient monitoring, nursing notes, scheduling nursing staff). What are the possible consequences of computer use in these areas?

9. Discuss the hospital information system (HIS). What are the various "levels" of this system? What is the role of the nursing department within this system?

10. Discuss the potential change associated with the introductionof computer use. What are the implications for the nurse manager?

CHAPTER 8

Motivating Staff

Chapter Outline

I. Why Motivate People?

II. What Motivates People?
   A. What energizes human behavior?
   B. What directs behavior?
   C. How is behavior sustained over time?

III. Content Theories of Motivation
   A. Instinct theories
      1. Freud
   B. Need hierarchy theories
      1. Maslow's need hierarchy
         a. Physiological needs
         b. Safety needs
         c. Belongingness or social needs
         d. Esteem needs
         e. Self-actualization
      2. Alderfer's ERG theory
         a. Existence needs
         b. Relatedness needs
         c. Growth needs
   C. Two-factor theory
      1. Extrinsic factors
      2. Intrinsic factors

IV. Process Theories of Motivation
   A. Reinforcement theory
      1. Operant conditioning
      2. Positive reinforcement
      3. Negative reinforcement
      4. Punishment
      5. Extinction
      6. Shaping
      7. Continuous schedule of reinforcement
      8. Partial schedule of reinforcement
      9. Fixed ratio reinforcement schedule
      10. Variable ratio reinforcement schedule
      11. Fixed interval reinforcement schedule
   B. Expectancy theory
      1. Expectancy theory versus reinforcement theory
      2. Components of expectancy theory
         a. Expectancy
         b. Instrumentality
         c. Valence

   C. Equity theory
      1. Components of equity theory

             a. Ratio of outcomes to inputs of
                focal person
             b. Ratio of outcomes to inputs of
                comparison other
             c. Perceived equity or perceived inequity
          D. Goal setting theory
             1. Three basic propositions
                a. Specific goals lead to higher performance
                   than general goals
                b. Specific, difficult goals lead to higher
                   performance than specific, easy goals
                   provided the goals are accepted
                c. Incentives only affect behavior if they
                   cause individuals to change their goals or
                   to accept goals that have been assigned to
                   them
             2. Research support of goal setting theory
             3. Participation and goal setting

   V.   Summary of Motivational Theories

  VI.   Managing Change
        A. Rules for introducing change

 VII.   Undesirable Jobs

VIII.   Job Design
        A. Job enlargement
        B. Job enrichment
        C. Core job dimensions
           1. Skill variety
           2. Task identity
           3. Task significance
        D. Principles of job redesign
        E. Barriers to job redesign

  IX.   Climate and Morale
        A. Types of climates in an organization
           1. Group norms
           2. Groupthink
           3. Morale

Topics for Discussion

1. Define content theory. Describe one or two content theories. How can these theories be applied to nurses' behavior?

2. Define process theory. How do process theories differ from content theories? How would the application of process theory differ from that of content theory (within nursing)?

3. Discuss the various process theories of motivation. What are the major propositions of each? How would you implement each of these theories in nursing? What problems may you encounter when trying to implement each theory?

4. Give examples of change within the health care organization. What rules may be used to enhance the change process? Use one example and apply the rules for introducing change.

5. What is job design? What is the difference between job enlargement and job enrichment? What are the components of Hackman and Oldham's model? Using a specific nursing unit, (e.g., intensive care, psychiatry) apply the Hackman and Oldham model.

CHAPTER 9

Leadership Skills

Chapter Outline

I.   Leadership Defined
     A. Influence on others
     B. Interpersonal process
     C. Informal leadership
     D. Formal leadership

II. Bases of Power
     A. Reward power
     B. Punishment
     C. Information power
     D. Legitimate power
     E. Expert power
     F. Referent power

III. Leadership: Personality, Behavior, or Style?
     A. Historical review
     B. Leadership styles

IV. Theories of Leadership
     A. The contingency model (Fiedler)
         1. Leadership styles
             a. Relationship-oriented
             b. Task-oriented
         2. Dimension of situation favorability
             a. Leader-member relations
             b. Task structure
             c. Position power
     B. Path-goal theory
         1. Forms of leadership behavior
             a. Supportive leadership
             b. Directive leadership
             c. Achievement-oriented leadership
             d. Participative leadership
     C. The normative model of decision participation
         1. Purpose of the model--help managers decide when
             to allow the staff to participate in decision
             making
         2. Characteristics that determine effectiveness
             of the decision
             a. Quality or rationality of the decision
             b. Acceptance or commitment of subordinates
                 to execute the decision effectively
         3. An abbreviated version of the model

V.   A Social Learning Approach to Leadership
     A. Introduction to social learning theory

B. The nurse manager as a role model
C. Pygmalion effect
1. Research evidence
2. Application to the nursing setting

VI. Building a Team
A. Climate of leadership and group interaction
B. Developing a supportive climate
C. Physical proximity of group
D. Managing the communication process

VII. Putting It All Together

Topics for Discussion

1. What is leadership? How does it differ from management?

2. What is power? Identify and describe several power bases. Describe how these bases may be used when the nursing department interacts with other organizational departments and in interactions within the nursing department.

3. Identify several theories of leadership. What are the major propositions of each? How does path-goal theory differ from Fiedler's contingency model? How does the normative model differ from path-goal theory and Fiedler's model?

4. What is social learning? Why should the nurse manager be concerned with role modeling? Recall an incident where you learned through the use of a role model. What is the Pygmalion effect?

5. Discuss the importance of a work team. How may such a group be developed and maintained?

CHAPTER 10

Stress and Time Management

Chapter Outline

   I. Nature of Stress
- A. Antecedents and consequences of stress
- B. Stress defined
- C. Stress in the workplace

  II. Role Conflict and Role Ambiguity
- A. Responses to stress overload
- B. Results of employee stress
- C. Coping responses

 III. Managing Stress
- A. Strategies for nurse managers
- B. Decreasing subordinates' stress
- C. Institutional strategies

  IV. Delegation
- A. Process of delegation
- B. What not to delegate

   V. Time Management
- A. Problems with time
- B. Goal setting
- C. Time analysis
- D. Setting priorities
- E. Control of interruptions
- F. Telephone calls
- G. Drop-in visitors
- H. Transition time

  VI. Summary

Topics for Discussion

1. Define stress.

2. Outline the sources of stress.

3. Discuss role ambiguity and role conflict

4. Outline the consequences of stress.

5. Discuss methods of managing stress, both by the manager for the subordinate and in one's own life.

6. Discuss institutional strategies for controlling stress.

7. What roles do objectives play in time management? How are these objectives related to those described in Chapter 3? What are the five major questions that must be answered during the process of organizing one's objectives?

8. When is time wasted? What are the major types of time wasters? How may each of these be decreased? Identify the major wasters of your time.

9. Identify the paper work associated with the nurse manager's job. What methods might be used so that this work is completed more effectively?

10. Define delegation. What are the benefits of delegating work to subordinates? What three concepts are the basis for effective delegation?

11. What two decisions must be made when delegating authority? What steps can be taken to assure effective delegation of authority? What should never be delegated? Why?

CHAPTER 11

Critical Thinking

Chapter Outline

I. Introduction
   A. Definition of critical thinking

II. Distinctions Between Problem Solving and Decision Making

III. Problem Solving Defined

IV. Problem Solving Methods
   A. Trial and error
   B. Experimentation
   C. Past experience
   D. Self-limiting

V. Problem Solving Process

VI. Decision Making Defined

VII. Decision Making Strategies
   A. Satisficing
   B. Optimizing

VIII. Decision Making Conditions
   A. Certainty
   B. Risk
   C. Uncertainty

IX. Decision Making Process

X. Stumbling Blocks to Creativity
   A. Personality
   B. Rigidity
   C. Preconceived Ideas

XI. Creativity in Decision Making
   A. Creative process
   B. Characteristics of creative persons
   C. Managing creativity in health care settings

Topics for Discussion

1. What are the steps of the problem solving process? Using a problem you experienced on the job, follow the steps of this process. Did you arrive at the same conclusion as you did on the job?

2. Identify and describe several methods of problem solving. In what nursing situations would each of these methods be most appropriate? Least appropriate? Why?

3. What are some potential obstacles to the problem solving process? How may each of these obstacles be overcome?

4. Why is creativity an important aspect of decision making? What are some of the characteristics of creative people? What can the nurse manager do to stimulate creativity ofdecision makers?

5. Under what conditions of probability may decisions be made? What methods or techniques may be used to improve decision making under these conditions of probability?

CHAPTER 12

Managing Groups

Chapter Outline

I. Introduction
   A. Definition of groups
   B. Group leadership

II. Group Processes
   A. Phases of group development
      1. Norms
      2. Group roles
      3. Status
   B. Communication in groups
   C. Group consequences
      1. Productivity
      2. Satisfaction
   D. Development and growth
   E. The nurse manager as leader

III. Group decision making
   A. Groupthink
   B. Dialectical inquiry
   C. Risky shift
   D. When to use groups
   E. Types of decision making groups

IV. Teams and Team-building

V. Managing Committees and Task Forces
   A. Preparation
   B. Conducting the first meeting
   C. General guidelines
   D. Leading meetings
   E. Managing subsequent meetings
   F. Completing the task force's report

VI. Summary

Topics for Discussion

1. What is a group? How do they form?

2. What is the difference between individual productivity and decision making and those of a group?

3. What dysfunctional attributes do groups develop?

4. Describe group decision making. What is groupthink?

5. What is team building? How is it done?

CHAPTER 13

Recruiting and Selecting Staff

Chapter Outline

I. Job Analysis
   A. Results of job analysis
      1. Identification of principal responsibilities and duties of a given job
      2. Identification of components of each duty
      3. Identification of personal qualifications needed to perform the job
   B. Job analysis techniques
      1. Supervisory conferences
      2. Critical incidents
      3. Work sampling
      4. Observation
      5. Interviewing
      6. Questionnaires
      7. Checklists

II. Recruitment
   A. Role of the nurse manager
   B. Elements of recruiting strategy
      1. Where to look
      2. How to look
      3. When to look
      4. How to sell the organization to potential recruits

III. Interviewing
   A. Objectives of the selection interview
   B. Principles for effective interviewing
      1. Planning the interview
      2. Responding to the applicant
      3. Eliciting information
      4. Giving information
      5. Processing information
   C. Staying within the law
      1. The impact of EEO law on selection procedures
   D. Preparing for the interview
      1. Review job requirements
      2. Review the application and the resume
      3. Write any specific questions
      4. Prepare the setting
   E. Developing structured interview guides
      1. Content is based on task analysis data
      2. Behavioral simulation exercises
      3. Benefits of the interview guide

   F. The interviewing process
      1. Open the interview

        a. Develop and maintain rapport
        b. Outline the discussion and set time limits
        c. Avoid making first impressions
    2. Obtain information
        a. Use a structured interview guide
        b. Take notes
        c. Type of questions and their specific use
    3. Giving information
        a. Realistic job previews
    4. Closing the interview
    5. Concluding the interview

IV. Deciding to Hire
    A. Steps in making a decision
        1. Weigh the qualities required for the job in
            order of importance
        2. Weigh the qualities desired based on
            reliability of the data
        3. Weigh job dimensions by trainability
        4. Compare data across individuals
    B. Interview reliability and validity
        1. Intrarater versus interrater reliability
        2. Research results
        3. Decreasing subjective judgment
    C. Testing for selection
        1. Aptitude tests
        2. Personality and interest inventories
        3. Work sample tests
    D. Education, experience, and physical exams
        1. Education and experience as work sample tests
        2. References and letters of recommendation
        3. Application forms
        4. Physical exam
    E. Assessment centers
        1. The assessment center process
        2. Essential elements of the assessment center
            technique

V. Validity and Legality in Hiring
    A. Importance of the validity of
        selection predictors
        1. Title VII of the Civil Rights Act
    B. The discrimination complaint process
    C. The validation procedure
        1. Empirical validation
            a. Concurrent validation
            b. Predictive validation
        2. Content validation

Topics for Discussion

1. Discuss the purpose of job analysis. Identify the various job analysis techniques. Discuss the pros and cons of each technique as used in nursing.

2. What are the elements of a recruiting strategy? How does each of these elements relate to the health care industry? Discuss the impact of communication on the recruitment process.

3. What are the objectives of the employment interviewer? What are the principles for the effective employment interview? Discuss the development and use of the structured interview guide in nursing. Discuss the interviewing process and identify the major steps.

4. Identify the various selection tools. How may these be used in the selection of nurses? What steps should be followed when making the decision to hire?

5. What are the legal issues of selection? What is reliability? What is validity?

CHAPTER 14

Staff Development and Patient Education

Chapter Outline

I. Training
    A. Needs assessment
    B. Planning and implementation
    C. Learning principles
        1. Readiness to learn
        2. Motivation to learn
        3. Conditions for practice
            a. Part versus whole
            b. Spaced versus massed
            c. Overlearning
        4. Transfer of training
            a. Similarity between training context and and job context
            b. Stimulus generalization
            c. Label major steps
            d. Identify general principles of behavior to be learned
    D. Memory span
        1. Short-term memory
        2. Long-term memory
        3. Facilities of memory span
            a. Rehearsal
            b. Grouping items
            c. Chunking
            d. Organization
    E. Social learning theory
        1. Reinforcement theory
        2. Development and verification of information
        3. Model of social learning
            a. Anticipated reinforcement
            b. Choose and observe a model
            c. Retention process
            d. Cognitive learning
            e. Behavior reproduction
            f. Contingent reinforcement for behavior
            g. New behavior
            h. Attitude change if behavior is consistently effective
    F. Adult education theory
        1. Self-concept
        2. Experience
        3. Readiness to learn
        4. Problem-centered time perspective
    G. Staff development
        1. Orientation
            a. Role of the training staff
            b. Role of the nursing previews

         c. Realistic job previews
         d. Socialization
      2. Preceptor model of staff orientation
         a. Role of the staff nurse/preceptor
         b. Role of the department of education
      3. Staff development methods
         a. Internal/on-the-job
         b. External/off-the-job
      4. Audiovisual techniques

   II. Evaluation
      A. Evaluative criteria
         1. Trainee reaction
         2. Learning
         3. Behavior change
         4. Organizational impact

   III. Patient Education
      A. Factors influencing patient education
      B. Barriers to teaching
         1. Lack of priority
         2. Lack of time
         3. Lack of communication
         4. Lack of knowledge and confidence
         5. Lack of training skill
         6. Lack of family involvement
         7. Lack of continuity
         8. Poor motivation
         9. Patient's physical condition
        10. Patient's psychosocial adaptation to illness
      C. The institution's education and training department
         1. Patient education
         2. Continuing education for the staff
      D. Record keeping and evaluation
         1. Legal implications of records
         2. Types of educational records

Topics for Discussion

1. Discuss the principles of learning. Why should each of these principles
    be considered when developing training interventions? Discuss social
    learning theory.

2. Discuss the importance of staff development. What is the role of the
    nursing manager in staff orientation? Describe on-the-job training. What
    are the key behaviors of on-the-job training? How can the nursing manager
    improve the effectiveness of on-the-job training?

3. What is the preceptor model of staff orientation? Discuss the roles of
    the preceptor. How does the department of education influence the
    preceptor concept?

4. Discuss the importance of the evaluation of training programs. Why is evaluation often ignored? Identify and discuss the four evaluative criteria. Relate each of these to the health care organization.

5. Discuss the need for patient education. What are the responsibilities of the nursing manager? What factors limit the effectiveness of patient education? Discuss how these limitations may be minimized.

CHAPTER 15

Enhancing Employee Performance

Chapter Outline

I. Introduction

II. A Model of Job Performance
   A. Employee motivation as a stimulus for performance
   B. Employee ability as a deterrent to performance
   C. Summary: job performance = f (motivation x ability)

III. Diagnosing Performance Problems
   A. A model

IV. Strategies for Intervention
   A. Day-to-day coaching
   B. Dealing with a rule violation

V. Chemical Dependency: A Performance Issue
   A. Identifying the chemically dependent nurse
   B. Strategies for intervention
   C. Reentry

VI. Summary

Topics for Discussion

1. What is drug dependence? How can it be handled in the work place?

2. What is codependence? Is it prevalent in nursing? What can be done about it in the work place?

3. How do you diagnose poor performance?

4. What is "coaching" and how is it used? What is its relationship to discipline?

CHAPTER 16

Performance Evaluation and Appraisal

Chapter Outline

    I. Assumptions
      A. One of the major reasons for performance reviews is to help employees improve their future performance
      B. The performance appraisal process is difficult, but one can become more skilled at it
      C. Very few persons like the performance appraisal form they are required to use
      D. In order to be effective in completing the formal, year-end review, one must carry out the day-to-day aspects of the performance appraisal process
      E. Supervisors always evaluate their employees' performance
      F. The prescriptions given in this chapter will notwork for approximately 5% of employees
      G. Performance appraisals may differ in content for each employee group but the process remains relatively stable

   II. Performance Appraisal Uses
      A. Performance appraisals as the basis of administrative decisions
      B: Performance appraisals and the Equal Employment Opportunity law

  III. Performance Appraisal and the Law
      A. Guidelines to decrease the likelihood of discriminatory findings

   IV. Performance Measurement Issues
      A. Evaluation philosophy
          1. Absolute versus comparative judgment
      B. Components to be evaluated
          1. Traits/personal characteristics
          2. Results/bottom line
          3. Behavioral criteria
          4. Combination of criteria

    V. Specific Evaluation Methods
      A. Traditional rating scales
          1. Scale characteristics
      B. Essay evaluation
      C. Forced distribution evaluation
      D. Behavior-oriented rating scales
          1. Developmental procedures
      E. Management by objectives
          1. Steps in management by objectives

   VI. Who Evaluates?
      A. The immediate supervisor

       B. Evaluation by a committee
       C. Peer ratings
       D. Self-evaluations
       E. Subordinate ratings

  XII. Disciplining Employees
       A. Communicating with the personnel department
       B. Fairness of the discipline process
           1. Clear communication of rules and regulations
           2. Develop a system of progressive penalties
           3. Establish an appeals process
       C. Guidelines for effective discipline
       D. Key behaviors for disciplining employees

  XIII. Some Rules of Thumb
       A. Go beyond the form
       B. Postpone the appraisal interview if necessary
       C. Don't be afraid to change an inaccurate rating

Topics for Discussion

1. How may the results of performance appraisal be used? What are the legal
    issues associated with the uses of performance appraisal? Discuss the
    guidelines which, if followed, increase the legal defensibility of the
    performance appraisal.

2. Identify and discuss the specific methods of evaluation. What are the
    strengths and weaknesses of each? Which is (are) most appropriate for
    nursing?

3. Identify those individuals who are potential evaluators. Who appears to
    be the most appropriate evaluator of the nurse's performance? Why?

4. There are several types of performance rating error. Identify and discuss
    each. How may these sources of error be lessened? Discuss the importance
    of documenting employee performance. Describe one method of
    documentation.

5. Discuss the performance appraisal interview. How does the
    evaluator/nursing manager prepare for the interview? What are the key
    behaviors of the evaluator/nursing manager for the performance appraisal
    interview?

6. Identify and discuss the key behaviors of day-to-day coaching. Why is
    day-to-day coaching important? When should the nursing manager use
    coaching rather than discipline? Identify and discuss the key behaviors
    of disciplining employees.

CHAPTER 17

Understanding and Managing Nurse Absenteeism and Turnover

Chapter Outline

I. Absenteeism
   A. The cost of absenteeism
   B. A model of employee attendance
      1. Voluntary versus involuntary absenteeism
      2. Steers and Rhodes model
         a. Ability to attend
         b. Motivation to attend
            1. Job satisfaction
            2. Pressure to attend
   C. Controlling absenteeism
      1. Indirect versus direct control
      2. Diagnosing the problem
         a. Factors affecting ability to attend
         b. Factors affecting motivation to attend
   D. Absenteeism policies
   E. A systems perspective

II. Turnover
   A. Measurement issues
   B: Voluntary versus involuntary turnover
   C. Consequences of turnover
      1. Undesirable consequences
      2. Desirable consequences
      3. Cost of turnover
   D. Model of employee turnover
      1. The nurse's perceived ease of movement
         a. Personal characteristics of the nurse
         b. Economic conditions
         c. Accessibility of other hospitals
      2. The nurse's perceived desire to move
         a. Existing job alternatives with current employer
         b. Job satisfaction
   E. Strategies for controlling nurse turnover
      1. Diagnose the problem
      2. Direct versus indirect strategies of control
   F. A systems perspective

Topics for Discussion

1. Discuss Steers and Rhodes model of attendance/absenteeism behavior. What are the two main variables of this model? What is the distinction between voluntary and involuntary absenteeism? What are some examples of costs of absenteeism in nursing?

2. Using Steers and Rhodes model, discuss how absenteeism may be controlled. Over which of the two major variables that affect absenteeism does the organization have more control? Discuss potential action the nursing manager may take to decrease absenteeism.

3. Identify and discuss the different types of turnover. From the organization's point of view, what are the consequences of each type of turnover?

4. Discuss the model of employee turnover developed by Heneman and others. What are the major variables? What direct and indirect turnover control measures are available to the nursing manager?

CHAPTER 18

Nursing Associations and Collective Bargaining

Chapter Outline

    I. Health Care Labor Relations
- A. Labor laws
- B. Special bargaining issues for hospitals
  1. 1974 health care amendments
     - a. Strikes
     - b. Negotiations
     - c. Occupations and bargaining units
- C. Effects of unionization in health care
  1. Wages
  2. Size of nursing staff
  3. Cost

    II. Why Individuals Join Unions
- A. Unionism and the economy
- B. Unionism as an attempt to control the labor market

    III. Nurses, Unions and Professional Associations
- A. A history of unions within the nursing profession
- B. Issues in representation
  1. Collective bargaining
  2. Supervisory personnel as members

    IV. The Nurse Manager's Role With a Unionized Staff
- A. Administration of the union contract
  1. Causes of grievances
     - a. Misunderstanding
     - b. Intentional contract violation
     - c. Symptomatic problems outside the scope of the labor contract
- B. The grievance process
  1. Steps
     - a. Informal discussion with immediate supervisor
     - b. First formal step--written request is given to immediate supervisor
     - c. Meeting is held--if results are unsatisfactory, a written appeal is submitted to nursing administrator
     - d. A second meeting is held--if results are unsatisfactory, a written appeal may be submitted
     - e. Arbitration is invoked when no suggested solution is acceptable

  2. Suggestions for handling grievances
     - a. Be courteous and respectful

b. Do not threaten or bluff
c. Do not withhold relevant facts
   or information
d. Do not exhibit internal disagreements
e. Expedite the process
f. Learn from your mistakes
g. Stay objective
h. Evaluate and anticipate the other party--
   develop a strategy
i. Utilize all resources possible
j. Never refuse to meet the grievant's
   representatives
k. Respond appropriately to the bargaining unit representative
   while he/she holds that role as well as the role of employee
l. Keep discussions unemotional--adjourn and
   reschedule if needed
m. Denial of a grievance by the superior or agent does not
   prohibit the employee'scontinued pursuit of the grievance
n. The contract is the sole determinant of
   what is fair
o. Be prepared to compromise within the
   framework of the contract
p. Know the strengths and weaknesses of
   both sides of the issue
q. While bargaining, think of future changes
   and needs
r. Pat formulas do not settle grievances
   or solve problems
s. Know your bottom line for compromise
t. Observe time limits
u. Carefully write all grievances
v. Be aware of your temperament and the other
   party's temperament when adjusting a
   grievance
w. Do not become overconfident
x. Get all the facts and information, witnesses, and
   documentation

3. Key behaviors of the grievance hearing
   a. Put the grievant at ease
   b. Listen openly and carefully
   c. Discuss the problem with him/her calmly and with an open
      mind
   d. Get his/her story straight
   e. Consider the grievant's viewpoint
   f. Avoid snap judgment
   g. Make an equitable decision

V. Legal Framework of Canadian Labor Relations
   A. Characteristics
      1. Purposes of labor legislation
      2. Collective bargaining rights

        3. Regulation of employer-employee relations
        4. Differences between U.S. and Canadian
           approaches to labor legislation
    B. The certification process
        1. Obtaining bargaining rights
        2. The role of labor boards
    C. Strike restrictions
        1. Legal restrictions
    D. Compulsory grievance arbitration
        1. Mandatory provisions for arbitration
        2. Lodging of appeals
    E. Union security
        1. The Rand formula

VI. Historical Review of Collective Bargaining By
Canadian Nurses
    A. Early unions and associations
    B. Relationships between professional associations
       and nurses' unions
        1. Independent nursing unions
        2. The use of liaison committees by unions and
           professional associations
        3. National Federation of Nurses' Unions

VII. Disputes Resolution and Emerging Issues
    A. The use of strikes and grievance arbitration
    B. Professional responsibility committees

Topics for Discussion

1. Discuss health care labor relations. Which hospitals are subject to jurisdiction under U.S. labor law? What are unfair labor practices? How do the 1974 Health Care Amendments influence union activity? Discuss how unionization has influenced health care.

2. Discuss the relationship between nursing professional associations and unions. What are the pros and cons associated with membership in each of these two organizations?

3. Discuss the grievance process. Review the suggestions for handling grievances. What are the key behaviors to be followed in the grievance hearing?

4. What is the role of the nurse manager with a unionized staff? Discuss the responsibilities of the nurse manager to the organization and to the staff.

5. What are the major differences between the Canadian and U.S. approaches to labor legislation? How may the nurse manager in a Canadian hospital behave with a unionized staff as compared to his/her American counterpart?

6. What is the history of collective bargaining by Canadian nurses? Discuss the relationship between professional nursing associations and unions.

CHAPTER 19

Budgeting and Resource Allocation

Chapter Outline

I.   Introduction

II. Planning and Control
    A. Planning
        1. Communication
        2. Coordination
    B. Controlling

III. Budgetary Concepts and Considerations
    A. Responsibility accounting
    B. Motivational aspects _reach goal_
    C. Budget period _1 yr - Quarterly_
    D. Zero-base budgeting _start from zero - each year_
    E. Flexible budgeting _changes in activity - pts - staff, equipment_

IV. The Operating Budget
    A. Units of service
    B. Capital expenditure budget
    C. Supply and expense budget
        1. Monitoring the supply and expense budget

V.   The Personnel Budget
    A. Relevant components
        1. Units of service
        2. Mix in patient acuity
        3. Required hours of nursing care
        4. Fixed and variable staffing
        5. Technological changes
        6. Changes in medical practice
        7. Regulatory requirements
        8. Support services
        9. Plans for next year
    B. Staffing patterns
    C. Position control
    D. The FTE budget
    E. Differentials and overtime
    F. Benefits
    G. Monitoring the personnel budget

Topics for Discussion

1. Identify the four types of budgets. What are the advantages and disadvantages of each? Identify those budget components with which the nursing manager is directly involved.

2. What factors influence personnel budget planning? How may the nursing manager identify the extent to which each of these factors may be affecting the budget? Discuss the process of personnel budget development. What factors are involved in developing a staffing pattern?

3. Discuss the supply and expense budget. What steps should be followed in the development of a supply and expense budget? How is this budget monitored?

4. What is the capital expenditure budget? What are two common criteria associated with the capital expenditure budget?

CHAPTER 20

Managing and Initiating Change

Chapter Outline

I. Climate for Change
   A. Change is inevitable
   B. DRGs
   C. Opportunities for nurses

II. Nurse as Change Agent
   A. Definition
   B. Internal or external

III. Change Within a Systems Framework
   A. Organizational equilibrium
   B. A macro view

IV. The Process of Change
   A. Environmental, systemwide, or unit based
   B. Problem solving approach

V. Selected Change Theories
   A. Lewin's Force-field Model
   B. Lippitt's Phases of Change
   C. Havelock's Model
   D. Roger's Diffusion of Innovations
   E. Summary
   F. Perspectives

VI. The Seven Steps to Planned Change: An Eclectic Approach
   A. Assessment
      1. Identify problem
      2. Collect data
      3. Analyze data
   B. Planning
      1. Plan the change
   C. Implementation
      1. Implement the change
   D. Evaluation
      1. Evaluate
      2. Stabilize

VII. Change Agent Strategies
   A. Power-coercive
   B. Empirical-rational
   C. Normative-reeducative

VIII. Change Agent Skills

IX. Handling Resistance

X. Politics of Change
   A. Exercises to stimulate creative thinking

Topics for Discussion

1. How does a nurse manager deal with change?

2. What are the inevitable changes the nurse manager will face in the future.

3. What is the change process. Discuss the 7 steps of change.

4. Discuss at least 3 theories of change.

5. Discuss the need for creativity in organizational change.

CHAPTER 21

Quality Assurance and Risk Management

Chapter Outline

I. Introduction to Risk Management
   A. Historical perspective
   B. Negligence
      1. Custodial
      2. Professional
   C. Components of risk management programs
      1. Patient and/or family incident review
      2. Employee and visitor safety

II. Quality Assurance
   A. Quality assurance process
      1. Setting standards
      2. Determining criteria
      3. Evaluating performance
      4. Making plans for change
      5. Follow-up
   B. Monitoring nursing care
      1. Nursing audit
      2. Peer review
      3. Utilization review
      4. Patient satisfaction

III. A Risk Management Program
   A. Purpose of the program
   B. Tasks of the program
      1. Identify potential risks
      2. Review present monitoring system
      3. Analyze characteristics of the incidents
      4. Review and appraise safety and risk
         aspects of patient care
      5. Monitoring relevant laws and codes
      6. Eliminate or reduce risk
      7. Review the work of other relevant committees
         when determining liability, prevention,
         or action
      8. Identify the need for educating patients,
         family and staff
      9. Evaluate the results of the program
      10. Provide periodic reports to relevant others
   C. Program members
      1. Risk manager
      2. Nursing representatives
      3. Medical staff
      4. Patient accounts representative
      5. Legal counsel (ex-officio)
      6. Others by invitation
   D. The risk manager

1. Schedules meetings and prepares agendas
2. Reviews incident reports daily
3. Monitors data collection mechanisms
4. Periodically visits high risk patients
5. Periodically summarizes litigation
6. Prepares monthly incident report summary
7. Participates in the development of staff education programs

IV. Nursing's Role in Risk Management
   A. Incident reports
      1. A process for reporting incidents
         a. Discovery--who reports
         b. Notification of risk manager
         c. Investigation by risk manager
         d. Consultation
         e. Action by the risk manager
         f. Recording and filing all information
   B. Some examples
      1. Medication errors
      2. Diagnostic procedures
      3. Medical-legal incident
      4. Patient or family attitude toward care

V. Role of the Nurse Manager
   A. Key behaviors for handling a complaint
      1. Listen openly
      2. Do not speak until the person has had his/her say
      3. Avoid reacting emotionally
      4. Ask for his/her expectation about a solution
      5. Explain what you can and cannot do to solve a problem
      6. Agree on specific steps to be taken and specific deadlines
   B. Documentation
   C. A caring attitude

VI. Evaluation of Risk Management
   A. The need to monitor and analyze incident reports
   B. Benefits of a risk management program

Topics for Discussion

1. What is risk management? What are the components of a risk management program? How is a risk management program developed? Who are the members of a risk management committee? What are the responsibilities of the risk manager? Discuss the risk management organization model.

2. What are the areas of high risk in a health care organization? Which of these areas involves the department of nursing? What is the role of nursing in risk management? Discuss the process for reporting incidents

and why nurses are reluctant to report incidents. What are some examples of risk incident?

3. What is the role of the nurse manager in the risk management system? How may the behavior of the nursing manager influence a risk incident? Discuss the key behaviors of handling a complaint. How does the attitude of the nursing manager influence the risk management system?

4. Discuss the importance of monitoring and analyzing incident reports. What are the benefits of a risk management program?

CHAPTER 22

Dealing With Conflict

<u>Chapter Outline</u>

    I. Importance of Conflict
       A. Positive aspects
       B. Negative aspects

   II. What is Conflict?
       A. Intrapersonal
       B. Interpersonal
       C. Intragroup
       D. Intergroup

  III. Competition vs. Conflict
       A. Disruptive conflict

   IV. Conflict Process Model
       A. Antecedent conditions
       B. Nature of goals and their importance to conflict
       C. Other antecedents
          1. Roles
          2. Scarce resources
          3. Value/beliefs
          4. Task interdependency
          5. Differentiation
          6. Verifying mechanisms

    V. Group Process
       A. Intragroup conflict
       B. Intergroup conflict
       C. Intraorganizational conflict

   VI. Communication Problems

  VII. Conflict Management
       A. Suppressing
       B. Withdrawing
       C. Smoothing
       D. Avoiding
       E. Forcing
       F. Competing
       G. Negotiating
       H. Collaborating
       I. Compromising
       J. Confrontating

 VIII. Group Conflict Resolution
       A. Win-lose
       B. Lose-lose
       C. Lose-win

IX. Personal Conflict Resolution Styles
    A. Friendly helper
    B. Toughbattler
    C. Compromiser
    D. Problem solver

X. Conflict Intervention
    A. Conflict resolution
    B. Basic rules
    C. Other conflict management techniques

Topics for Discussion

1. What is conflict? Using Filley's model of conflict resolution, describe the conflict process specific to the nurse manager. What are antecedent conditions? What behaviors may be observed? Describe conflict resolution and conflict suppression.

2. How do factors such as role conflict and intraprofessional decisiveness lead to conflict for nurses? What other factors influence conflict in nursing?

3. How may conflict be managed? Discuss both effective and ineffective modes of response. Identify and describe three types of conflict outcomes and their respective strategies. Identify a situation where each strategy would be advantageous for the nursing manager.

4. Describe the conflict intervention process. When should intervention be avoided? What rules should the nurse manager follow when acting as a mediator? Why are these rules important?

5. What is stress? What are potential sources of stress for a nurse? What are the physiological and psychological responses to stress overload? Discuss both personal and institutional strategies for coping with stress.

CHAPTER 23

Power and Politics

Chapter Outline

I. Introduction

II. A Framework for Political Action
    A. Spheres of influence
    B. Political influence on health care
    C. Political influence on nursing care
    D. Participation in health care policies

III. Politics: The Art of Influencing
    A. Allocation of resources
    B. An interpersonal endeavor
    C. A collective endeavor
    D. Analysis and planning
    E. Effective political action

IV. Using Power to Increase Professional Influence
    A. The concept of power
    B. Types of power
    C. The perception of power
    D. Nurses' need for power

V. Marketing: Image as Power
    A. Perception by others
    B. Promoting an image of power
    C. Professional concern with images of power
    D. Marketing professional expertise and ability

IV. Summary

Topics for Discussion

1. What is "power"? What is "politics"? How are they related? How should they be used by nurses?

2. How do nurses gain power? How do they gain and use power in organizations?

3. How do nurses use the political process overall? In organizations?

4. What should nurses do to gain more power, status and responsibility in the health care system?

CHAPTER 24

A Pragmatic View of Nursing Management

Chapter Outline

     I. Introduction

    II. Transition

   III. Socialization For The Role of Nurse Manager

    IV. Identification With Management

     V. Career or Job?

    VI. Politics

   VII. Knowing The System

 VIII. Keeping Up With Trends
   A. Social trends
   B. Health care trends
   C. Nursing trends

    IX. Colleagues, Mentors, and Sponsors
   A. Colleagues
      1. Definition
      2. Development of colleagueship
   B. Mentors
      1. Definition
      2. Stages of mentor/protege relationships
         a. Initiation stage
         b. Protege stage
         c. Breakup stage
         d. Lasting friendship stage
      3. Hazards of a mentor relationship
      4. Suggestions for examining a toxic relationship
      5. Self-mentors
   C. Sponsors
      1. Description
      2. Rules for mentor or sponsor relationships

     X. Groups
   A. Hints for leading group discussions

    XI. Basic Survival Skills

   XII. The First Weeks as Manager
   A. First day on the job
   B. Meeting and dealing with staff
   C. Initial staff meetings
   D. Strengthening your position in the early weeks

E. Dealing with insecurities

XIII. Strategies For Working With Your Boss
A. Managing upward
B. Other strategies for managing your boss
C. Influencing your boss
D. Taking a problem to your boss

XIV. Working With Physicians

Topics for Discussion

1. How is authority conceptualized within the hospital system? What is power? What are the formal and informal power structures within the health care organization? How may the use of formal power structures differ from the use of informal power structures? How may the nursing manager develop informal power?

2. What characteristics of the subordinate influence the superior/subordinate relationship? What are the responsibilities of the subordinate in the superior/subordinate relationship? Identify several basic principles for working with superiors; why are these principles important?

3. Discuss the importance of the subordinate's preparing his/her request of the superior. What should the subordinate consider before making a request? What are the key behaviors for a subordinate when taking a problem to the superior? What are the advantages of using these key behaviors?

4. Discuss the factors that may influence the nurse/physician interaction. What are the implications for the nurse manager?

5. Identify three general areas to monitor for trends. What is the impact of each of these areas on nursing?

6. What is power? How can a nursing manager develop effective political power? Imagine your work situation; how would you go about developing your power?

7. Discuss the role of a mentor. How does this compare with the role of a sponsor? Discuss the rules for the mentor or sponsor relationship.

8. Identify several of the key behaviors for successful nursing management. If you are a nursing manager, critique your performance using these key behaviors or critique a nursing manager with whom you are familiar.

SECTION II

◊

TESTBANK

CHAPTER 1 - INTRODUCTION TO NURSING MANAGEMENT

TRUE/FALSE:

1. There are currently over 30 million Americans in the United States who work, but are inadequately covered by insurance.

2. By the year 2000, it is expected that 33 percent of the United States population will be over 65 years of age and 5 percent will be over the age of 85.

3. Acute diseases are now the primary condition for which our society seeks health care.

4. It is predicted that the current nursing shortage will end in the near future.

5. It has been found that nurses who have input into decisions about their work were more satisfied and remained in their positions longer.

6. Nurse managers and their staff may demonstrate codependent tendencies.

7. In an ideal nursing structure, there should only be the nurse manager between the one top nursing executive and the staff.

8. Manipulative communication is productive to team building.

9. The first step in effective communication is listening.

Answers:

1) True, p. 4	6) True, p. 8
2) False, p. 5	7) True, p. 9
3) False, p. 5	8) False, p. 9
4) False, p. 5	9) True, p. 9
5) True, p. 7	

MULTIPLE CHOICE:

10. Key issues that will influence and create change in the delivery of health care in our society in the near future center are: (pp. 4-5)

    a.   the economics of health care
    b.   the competitive nature of the industry
    c.   the shortages of professional healthcare workers
    d.   the focus on quality outcomes and consumerism
  * e.   all of the above

11. During the nursing shortage, the greatest need will be for which type of nurse? (p. 5)

a. nurses prepared at the associate degree level
b. nurses prepared at the baccalaureate level
* c. nurses prepared at the masters level

12. According to Block, empowerment stems from which sources? (p. 8)

   a. from the structure, practices and policies we support as
      managers who have control over others
   b. personal choices we make that are expressed by our own actions
   c. managers who possess codependent tendencies
* d. a and b
   e. c only

13. Effective communication strategies that support and build team
    commitment are all of the following <u>except</u>: (p. 9)

   a. listening
   b. being forthright about what is needed
   c. directing communications to the correct party
* d. the use of manipulative communication

14. Nurse managers are accountable to ensure that the patient's expectations
    of care are met. The first step in improving customer service is to:
    (p. 6)

   a. establish standards of performance
* b. identify customer expectations
   c. train staff to meet expectations

15. How many Americans in the United States who work are inadequately
    covered by health insurance? (p. 4)

   a. 10 million
   b. 20 million
* c. 30 million
   d. 40 million

16. According to Statland, what will ascend to be the leading health care
    issue in the 1990's? (p. 5)

   a. cost
   b. technology
* c. quality of health care

17. Which of the following are ways to identify patient expectations of
    nursing care? (p. 6)

   a. surveys
   b. focus groups
   c. nursing rounds
* d. all of the above
   e. a only

18. Discuss key issues for health care in the 1990's that will influence and create change in the delivery of health care in our society in the future.

   The major issues focus on health care economics, the competitive nature of the industry, the shortage of professional health care workers and the focus on quality care outcomes and consumerism. These changes will necessitate new and different leadership for nurse managers in the future. They must be flexible, intelligent and possess new leadership expertise. Managers must focus on productivity as a way to reduce costs. They need strong financial skills in budgeting and cost variance reporting. Nurse managers must also be well versed in information technologies, staff retention and recruitment as well as staff development. (p. 1-6)

19. Discuss key issues for nurse managers in the 1990's.

   Managers at all levels must assess their organizational missions and the changes that are occurring in their environment to ensure that they are defining a vision for their work groups. The work group can, therefore, establish the standards, systems and processes that will result in quality patient care. The manager facilitates the development of standards and role models' behaviors that support them. Managers must allow the professional to be autonomous in the delivery of care. Managers with codependent tendencies must recognize these behaviors and make efforts to change this behavior. Managers should support failure and publicly reward mistakes. Managers must be effective communicators with all members of the organization. (p. 6-9)

20. Define characteristics of codependents according to Cauthorne-Lindstrom and Hrabe. (p. 8)

   Powerful need to take care of others
   Rigidity and perfectionism
   Difficulty adjusting to changes
   Need to control situations and people
   Denial or distortion of anger
   Secret feeling of powerlessness
   Dependence on others for approval
   A basic sense of shame or poor self concept

21. Discuss how decentralization of decision making and empowerment can work effectively.

   Members of the organization must be able to take risks and the organization must develop a culture where risk taking is rewarded and failure is accepted. Managers must assure staff that mistakes are expected and that human error is inevitable. (p. 9)

22. Discuss effective communication strategies that support and build team commitment.

    Listening is the first strategy, especially empathetic listening which is to understand where others are and what they need. Listening is the first and most important step in communication. Secondly, managers must have the courage to be forthright about what is needed from others. Thus, it is important to clearly articulate expectations. The third strategy is to communicate directly to the individual who needs to hear the information and receive feedback. Nurse managers must expect direct communication from staff and role model this behavior so that it will become a standard for the group. (p. 9-10)

23. Discuss what impact that the focus on quality health care in the 1990's will have on nurse managers.

    It will require that nurse managers learn new ways to measure quality and new approaches in the evaluation of systems that result in quality care. They will also need to acquire new problem solving techniques to ensure that those involved in health care services are committed to the continuous improvement of services. (p. 2-3)

CHAPTER 2 - The Nature of Organization in Health Care

TRUE/FALSE

1. Continuously working together under authority toward a goal implies management.

2. The most common way modern organizational theorists analyze organizations is through a systems perspective.

3. The optimal organizational structure integrates organizational goals, size, technology, and environment.

4. The largest number of health care organizations in this country today are long term care institutions.

5. Shared governance is a system that allows the staff nurse an equal vote in major decisions about nursing practice.

6. It is a simple task to define organizational effectiveness in a service industry such as health care.

7. Most bureaucratic organizations are thought to be very effective.

8. Health care today is viewed in a stable, predictable environment.

Answers:

1.	True,	p. 12	5.	True,	p. 33
2.	True,	p. 13	6.	False,	p. 35
3.	True,	p. 22	7.	False,	p. 17
4.	False,	p. 30	8.	False,	p. 22

MULTIPLE CHOICE

9. In order to describe the structure of an organization, which of the following macro components need <u>not</u> be included? (p. 13)

    a. complexity
  * b. budget
    c. formalization
    d. centralization

10. Which of the following is an untrue statement regarding systems? (p. 13)

    a. A system is a set of interrelated parts arranged in a unified whole.
    b. Societies, automobiles, human bodies and hospitals are viewed as systems.
  * c. All systems are classified as "open".

d. The open system perspective recognizes the interaction of the system with its environment.

11. Which of the following theories is not considered to be a result or a view of organizational theory? (p. 15-18)

   a. classical theory
   b. neoclassical theory
 * c. path goal theory
   d. technological theory
   e. modern systems theory

12. According to the neoclassical theorists, classical theory failed to recognize which of the following elements? (p. 17)

 * a. the motivation of the individual
   b. the division and specialization of labor
   c. the chain of command
   d. the structure of the organization
   e. the span of control

13. Woodward, the technological theorist, categorized firms into all of the following types of technology except: (p. 18)

   a. unit (custom-made products)
   b. mass (large batch manufacturing)
 * c. systems (input, output, throughput)
   d. process production (continuous process manufacturing)

14. All of the following are considered to be modern systems theorists except: (p. 18-19)

   a. Katz and Kahn
   b. March and Simon
 * c. Frederick Taylor
   d. Galbraith

15. Most organizations fall within one of the following structures except: (p. 25-30)

   a. functional structure
   b. hybrid structure
   c. self-contained unit structure
 * d. task structure
   e. matrix structure

16. Health care organizations can be typically categorized in all of the following ways except: (p. 30-31)

   a. acute care institutions
   b. long term care institutions
   c. home health care agencies

d. temporary health care services
* e. medical emergency centers

17. Which of the following statements are not true regarding shared governance? (p. 33)

   a. allows the staff nurse a vote in decisions about nursing practice
   b. usually built on a foundation of primary nursing, peer review and provision for clinical advancement
   c. most shared governance systems are designed along the lines of academic or medical governance models
   * d. patient care generally diminishes when nurses control their own practice

18. Three key variables in classic organization theory are: (p. 15-16)

   a. span of attention, span of control, and structure
   b. span of control, structure, and need hierarchy
   * c. span of control, specialization, and delegation of authority
   d. delegation of authority, specialization, and goal clarity

19. On the basis of the research of Joan Woodward, one would conclude that: (p. 18)

   a. delegation of authority is a matter of preference
   b. structure depends solely on the number of people employed by an organization
   c. specialization inhibits goal clarity
   * d. span of control is related to technology

20. The major difference between classic and modern approaches to organization theory is: (p. 15-20)

   a. the structure of the organization
   * b. the introduction of human emotions
   c. the size of the organization
   d. the effects of outside forces
   e. all of the above

21. Span of control refers to: (p. 15-16)

   * a. the number of subordinates controlled by a single supervisor
   b. those people who have direct responsibility for goods and services
   c. those people who serve in an advisory capacity
   d. none of the above

22. Which of the following is not a component of classic organization theory? (p. 16)

   a. span of control

b. structure
c. division of labor
d. delegation of authority
* e. all of the above are components of this theory

ESSAY QUESTIONS

23. Outline at least eight characteristics that are common to all open systems. (p. 12-13)

   a. input or impartation of energy
   b. throughput
   c. output
   d. system of cyclic events
   e. negative entropy
   f. information input
   g. steady state
   h. differentiation
   i. integration/coordination
   j. equifinality

24. Define contingency theory and list the forces that assist in achieving optimal organization performance. (p. 22)

   Definition - Contingency theory is that part of organization theory which seeks to establish a set of general principles for matching an organization's structure most closely to the forces of the environment, technology, people, and goals to achieve optimal organizational performance.

25. Discuss organizational structures unique to health care. (p. 30)

   Typically, the medical staff is separate and autonomous from the organization, which results in an organizational dilemma: two lines of authority. One line extends from the governing body to the CEO and then to the managerial structure. The other line extends from the governing body to the medical staff. The two lines intersect in departments such as nursing in which decision making contains both managerial and clinical elements. Hospitals with a functional structure and separate medical governance are referred to as parallel structures.

26. Discuss the various elements that must be present to achieve organizational effectiveness for health care institutions. (p. 35-36)

   1. Adaptability - the ability to solve problems in reaction to a changing environment.
   2. A sense of organizational purpose - a sharing by all members of the organization of knowledge and insight as to where an organization is headed and why.
   3. Ability to test reality - the ability to search out, perceive and

interpret the environment and implications for the organization.
4. Integration - the ability to ensure that all organizational subparts are integrated and not working at cross purposes.

CHAPTER 3 - THE FUNCTIONS OF A NURSE MANAGER IN HEALTH CARE SETTINGS

TRUE/FALSE

1. From a broad perspective, management can be viewed not only as the process of getting work done through others, but can also include planning, staffing, organizing, directing, controlling and decision making.

2. Planning is a three-stage process consisting of establishing objectives, formulating a planning statement and converting this into an action statement.

3. Without clear cut goals, health care institutions spend a disproportionate amount of their time "fighting fires" instead of in "fire prevention".

4. French and Raven classified sources of power into five categories: reward, coercive, legitimate, expert and referent power.

5. Patient care is organized according to the type of delivery system used. The basic types of care are functional, team and primary nursing, case management and differentiated practice.

Answers:

1) True, p. 39   4) True, p. 48
2) False, p. 39-41   5) True, p. 47
3) True, p, 42

MULTIPLE CHOICE

Situation 1

Ms. Alexander has recently been hired for a first-line management position on a 38 bed neuro unit. She is a baccalaureate graduate who has worked as a staff nurse for the past three years in another hospital. She has had no previous management experience. Ms. Alexander is aware that she needs to acquire additional knowledge and experience if she is to become an effective manager. (Figure 3-1, p. 44)

6.   Ms. Alexander needs more specific knowledge and skills in the area of task technology which would include understanding of: (Fig. 3-1, p. 40)

          a. legal-governmental processes
    *   b. work design
          c. communication
          d. ecology

7.   Another important managerial area in which Ms. Alexander needs additional knowledge and practice is how to manage people. This would

include all of the following areas of information <u>except</u>: (Figure 3-1, p. 44)

    a. learning style
    b. motivation
    c. values
* d. span of control

<u>Situation 2</u>

Ms. Alexander is now responsible for the management functions of organizing, planning, controlling, and decision making on her unit. These activities comprise many subcomponents or specific interventions.

8. The priority activity involved in the planning process is which of the following? (p. 41)

    a. identification of product and services
* b. setting unit objectives
    c. establishing efficiency criteria of work performance
    d. predicting and evaluating

9. The priority activity involved in the organizing process is: (p. 47-48)

* a. mobilizing material and human resources
    b. comparing results with predetermined standards
    c. taking corrective action if performance deviates from the set standard

10. Planning represents management's attempt: (p. 39)

    a. to anticipate the future
    b. to alleviate anxiety about the future
    c. to visualize the future
* d. to determine in advance what to do in the future
    e. all of the above

11. The steps involved in control include which of the following: (p. 49)

    a. establishing standards of performance
    b. determining methods of measuring performance
    c. evaluation of the performance
    d. feedback of performance data
    e. all of the above except d
* f. all of the above

12. Planning includes all of the following <u>except</u>: (p. 39)

    a. establishing objectives
    b. evaluating the present situation and predicting

future trends
* c. mobilizing human and material resources
d. formulating a planning statement

13. Institutional objectives can be categorized into four areas.
They are: (p. 41)

* a. services, efficiency, social and human resources
b. patients, medical staff, other staff, and community
c. products, services, facilities, and community
d. resources, efficiency, budgeting, governmental agencies

14. Goal displacement is described as: (p. 45)

a. pursuing narrow unit goals rather than overall hospital goals
b. excessive enforcement of unit rules rather than those of
the institution
c. none of the above
* d. both a and b

15. The most important means of coordination is the _____
of institutions. (p. 47)

a. control systems
b. sources of power
c. performance appraisal system
* d. authority structure

16. Anticipatory socialization is best defined as: (p. 50)

a. learning in a presocializing institution like a
school of nursing
b. learning the norms and values of an organization
* c. acquiring what one believes to be the attitudes, values or
beliefs of the group one hopes to join
d. being accepted into full membership status in an institution
e. none of the above

17. Managerial surveillance is: (p. 50)

a. direct observation of subordinate behavior
b. indirect observation through records
c. narrowing span of control in order to better supervise
d. all of the above
* e. a and b

18. March & Simon have pointed out that many decision makers tend to
use _____ most often. (p. 52)

a. optimizing
* b. satisficing

72

    c. the Delphi technique
    d. decision making under uncertainty

19. MBO is most effective in increasing employee: (p. 49)

    a. moral
    b. satisfaction
    c. productivity
  * d. a and b
    e. b and c

ESSAY QUESTIONS

20. What is the importance of setting objectives? How would the absence of objectives in each of the four general areas (e.g., product/service) influence the nursing department? Present and discuss examples of objectives specific to nursing.

    a. to focus thinking on the future, to be proactive, to plan (short-term and long-term), to do contingency planning, to avoid goal displacement, to involve all organizational members, and to aid evaluation/prediction of future events.
    b. strategic/contingency planning, prediction and evaluation of service in each area cannot occur without objectives
    c. see text for examples (p. 41).

21. Describe the process of socialization. Using an example relevant to nursing, describe the movement through the five stages of this process. What are the implications for nursing management?

    a. stages of socialization:
        a. anticipatory socialization
        b. learning in a presocializing institution
        c. recruitment
        d. institutional socialization
        e. "rite of passage"
    b. example
    c. look for facilitating the process of socialization, understanding the universal nature of the process, and understanding the role transformation from student to nurse (pp. 49-50).

22. Discuss the relationship between the planning process and organizational structure.

    Look for types of planning (strategic, contingency, or operational), organizational level in planning, goal congruence both vertically and horizontally and a connection between planning and evaluation (pp. 42-46)

23. Identify methods of organizing or coordinating (e.g., authority and power) and discuss the implications for nursing management (e.g., scheduling staff, training personnel).

        a. methods:
             authority
             power
             departmentalization
             bureaucracy
        b. implications
             scheduling
             staffing
             training
             appraising
             nursing delivery system (p. 47-49)

24.   Describe six management functions described in Chapter 3.

          planning
          staffing
          organizing
          directing
          controlling
          decision making (p. 39)

25.   What are the factors affecting the nurse manager? Name examples of
      each.

          See Figure 3-1, p. 40

26.   Describe Management by Objectives (MBO).

      A process in which the overall objectives of the organization are
      disseminated down into the organization so that each individual is
      involved. The process includes identifying objectives and showing
      these to department heads, who then formulate objectives for each
      unit. These are discussed to insure congruence. Each subordinate
      works on developing a plan to achieve the goals. Measures of
      achievement are predetermined and feedback is given to each
      subordinate.
      (p. 49)

27.   Describe the four phases in the role transformation from student to
      staff nurse as explicated by Schmalenberg & Kramer (1979).

          honeymoon phase
          shock
          recovery
          resolution (p. 50)

28.   Compare and contrast the tasks of the clinical nurse and nurse manager
      within the framework of assessment-planning-implementation-evaluation.

          See Figure 3-6, p. 55

74

29.   Discuss the importance of authority in the process of coordination.
      Make sure you discuss the two types of authority rights and sources of
      power.

      a. the most important means of coordination includes the right to
         allocate tasks and to evaluate performance. Sources of power
         include: reward, coercive, legitimate, expert, and referent
         (pp. 50-51)

CHAPTER 4 - ORGANIZING CARE

<u>TRUE/FALSE</u>

1. A key factor that distinguishes case management from other systems of nursing care delivery is the case manager's accountability for care coordination that transcends unit and service boundaries.

2. Functional nursing is the most popular and utilized system of nursing care delivery.

3. The original form of nursing care delivery was team nursing.

4. Staffing is probably the most pressing issue facing nursing leaders.

5. The Joint Commission on Accreditation of Healthcare Organizations requires that staffing levels be based on a determination of patient acuity.

6. An advantage of computerized scheduling is individualizing the needs of the staff.

7. The purpose of patient classification systems is to provide an objective format for determination of workload requirements.

8. Adoption of a patient classification system is seldom costly.

Answers:

1)	True, p. 62	5)	True, p. 67
2)	False, p. 64	6)	False, p. 71
3)	False, p. 64	7)	True, pp. 69-70
4)	True, p. 66	8)	False, p. 70

<u>MULTIPLE CHOICE</u>

9. All of the following are models of differentiated practice <u>except</u>: (p. 62)

   * a. nursing process based
     b. education based
     c. assessment based
     d. all professional

10. Which of the following statements <u>least</u> accurately describes the case management method of nursing care delivery? (p. 62)

    a. developed in response to a need for more effective coordination of patient care
    b. a method whereby the professional nurse maintains responsibility from admission through and following discharge
    c. the case manager's accountability for care coordination

transcends unit and service boundaries
* d. designed to place the registered nurse back at the bedside

11. Which statement is <u>not</u> true regarding team nursing? (p. 64)

    a. it is used by a majority of U.S. hospitals
    b. it is the delivery of care by nursing staff of various
       educational preparations
* c. it implies 24 hour accountability for client care
    d. team members provide direct patient care under the supervision
       of the team leader
    e. the team leader is responsible for communicating with
       physicians, allied health personnel and resolving problems
       encountered by the team members

12. Which of the following statements best describe functional nursing care delivery? (p. 64)

    a. commonly practiced in the 1950's in response to a
       national nursing shortage
    b. continues to be used in the majority of hospitals today
    c. nursing tasks are divided with one nurse responsible for
       medications, another treatments, and another baths
* d. a and c
    e. b

13. Various approaches to solve problems of nursing staffing may be the utilization of: (p. 69)

    a. nursing staff agencies
    b. float pools
    c. nurse extender roles
* d. all of the above
    e. a and b only

14. Some advantages of using patient classification systems are: (p. 70)

    a. to provide an objective format for determination
       of workload requirements
    b. to provide tracking of information for budgeting and
       productivity analyses

    c. to serve as care plans and costing out nursing care.
    d. a and b only
* e. all of the above

15. Which of the following is not a patient classification system? (p. 71, Table 4-4)

* a. PERT
    b. GRASP

77

        c. MEDICUS
        d. ARIC
        e. Riverside

16.   Which is the most utilized patient classification system in U.S.
       hospitals? (p. 71, Table 4-4)

        a. self-deficit
        b. Riverside
     * c. MEDICUS
        d. GRASP
        e. ARIC

ESSAY QUESTIONS

17.   Discuss the major concepts and purpose of product line management as
       applied to the hospital setting. (p. 65)

           The project manager is held accountable for production efficiency,
           marketing and product outcome, and is empowered to make necessary
           decisions to affect product success. As applied to health care
           product line management requires the definition of "products" such
           as rehabilitation, women's health or arthritis care. Specific
           areas of service needs are identified for targeted marketing. The
           product manager maintains accountability for cost effective
           "production" of the service.

18.   Describe the primary nursing delivery system of care. (pp. 62-63)

           The underlying principle of primary nursing is that the registered
           nurse maintains a caseload of "primary" patients for whom the nurse
           designs, implements, and is accountable for the nursing care plan.
           Primary nursing enables nurses to directly complete the patient
           care for which they were educated without the need to delegate care
           or supervise non-professional staff. The primary nurse is
           accountable on a 24 hour a day basis to the patient and for their
           nursing care plan.

19.   List three disadvantages or problems of team nursing. (p. 64)

       1. The limited amount of time the team leader spends with the
          patients; thus, more communication and information about the
          patient comes from the team members.
       2. Possible role confusion and resentment. Team members sometime
          view the role of team leader as more focused on paperwork and
          less focused on patient needs.
       3. Problems in communication and delegation with so many team members.

20.   Discuss JCAHO accreditation requirements for staffing. (p. 67-70)

Requires that staffing levels be based on a determination of patient acuity. The JCAHO survey/review staffing levels to determine if such levels are sufficient for:
    patient care requirements
    staff expertise
    unit geography
    support services
    method of patient care delivery
JCAHO does not identify a specific level of nursing care hours.

21.   List five goals of staffing. (p. 66)

    a. to project patient care needs
    b. to evaluate the level of quality provided
    c. to provide the number and mix of nursing staff needed
    d. to anticipate the availability of nursing staff
    e. to provide low cost, high quality nursing care

CHAPTER 5 - PRODUCTIVITY

TRUE/FALSE

1. The diagnostically-related groups (DRGs) payment system classifies patients into resource-use groups based on their diagnosis, age and the use of certain procedures; each group is then assigned an average cost for patient care.

2. Nursing productivity is clearly defined as a function of its inputs, processes and outputs; each of these components can be readily defined and measured.

3. Jelinek and Dennis proposed a model for evaluating nursing productivity based on a systems approach which showed the relationship between inputs, processes and outputs and which suggested the consideration of environmental influences on the three elements.

4. Currently, resources per patient day, degree of occupation and utilization rates are used to measure nursing productivity.

5. Nursing productivity may be improved primarily by changing the environment in which the services are performed.

Answers:

    1) True, p. 80
    2) False, pp. 81-83
    3) True, p. 81
    4) True, pp. 82-85
    5) False, p. 87

MULTIPLE CHOICE

Situation 1

Mary Ann Adams, the nurse manager or an adult medical unit of 38 beds, is researching methods of measuring nursing productivity in order to determine the most effective and efficient method for her unit.

6. Mary Ann knows the best definition of nursing productivity as related to health care delivery is: (p. 81)

    a. the relationship between the output of an industry and the resources required to produce that output
    b. the ratio between the dollar value of the inputs (hours of labor, equipment, etc.) to the dollar return on the outputs (patient days)
  * c. the relationship between input, processes, and output as determined by the quality and the quantity of the output.

7. Mary Ann is presently using the method of nursing hours per client day

to determine performance productivity. This method is limited because it measures one single input. That input is: (p. 83)

    a. the acuity of the client
    b. the skill level and mix of nursing staff
  * c. the number of hours of nursing care
    d. the quality of the patient days being produced

8.   All of the following statements are true concerning the degree-of-occupation method of measuring nursing productivity <u>except</u>: (p. 84)

    a. the nurse manager utilizes an informal busyness scale to determine degree to which staff is occupied
    b. the nurse manager makes a judgment as to whether the number of staff members is sufficient to handle the work load each day
    c. the degree of occupation of the staff can be determined by the activity on the unit that day (e.g., admissions, transfers, discharges, patient teaching)
  * d. the nurse manager utilizes a patient classification system to determine degree of staff occupation

9.   Mary Ann has determined that she and her staff can improve nursing productivity by instituting changes in the use of inputs. This would include all of the following <u>except</u>: (pp. 87-88)

    a. matching supply with demand
    b. making staff substitutions
  * c. measuring outcome
    d. controlling the use of supplies and equipment

10.   Resources per patient day and degree of occupation are: (pp. 83-84)

    a. methods of ordering supplies
  * b. measures of nursing productivity
    c. nursing DRG's
    d. staffing schedules

11.   Which of the following is <u>not</u> a method of increasing productivity? (pp. 87-90)

    a. controlling use of supplies
    b. making staff substitutions
    c. matching supply and demand
  * d. giving the staff the Position Analysis Questionnaire

12.   According to the text, which method of increasing productivity allows the nurse manager to use her/his creativity to the fullest? (p. 90)

  * a. changes in the care process
    b. controlling use of supplies and equipment
    c. making staff substitutions
    d. matching supply with demand

13. One of the best known performance measures used in nursing is: (pp. 85-86)

    a. ratio of expected to required staff levels
  * b. ratio of required to actual staffing levels
    c. documentation flow sheets
    d. product-line unit-cost performance

14. Sovie suggests all the following as productivity enhancement strategies except: (pp. 89-90)

    a. generic care plans
    b. separate nursing charges from room charges
    c. develop new products
  * d. reuse old products

ESSAY QUESTIONS

15. Discuss the need for productivity measurement and improvement in nursing service today.

    Nursing is the largest group of health providers and largest cost-center in a hospital. Nursing is not billed separately and nursing services are ill-defined. (p. 79)

16. Outline the differing methods of measuring productivity.

    a. Resources per patient day
    b. Degree of occupation
    c. Utilization rates required to actual staffing (pp. 83-86)

17. Compare and contrast the different attempts to define productivity in health care.

    Look for discussion of inputs vs. outcomes, the nature of the product, how outcomes are measured, and measurement of quality (p. 81)

18. Discuss the nature of a hospital's input and output in the measurement of productivity.

    Inputs = labor, materials, equipment used in production of service (they usually can be measured)
    Outcome = nursing service, case-mix measures, quality of service (very difficult to measure)
    Look for opinion on quality vs. quantity (pp. 81-87)

19. What is nursing productivity?

    ratio of output per input adjusted by quality and safety
        resources per patient day
        degree of occupation

utilization rates (p. 81)

20. How would one approach improving nursing productivity?

    a. changes in uses of inputs
        match supply with demand
        make staff substitutions
        control use of supplies
    b. changes in care process
        work schedules
        nursing rituals
        delivery system
    c. documenting savings (pp. 87-90)

21. Define productivity. Discuss methods of measuring it.

    a. see Question #20
    b. see Question #17

22. Discuss methods to improve nursing productivity.

    See #17, look for a distinction between changes in use of inputs and changes in care process. Look for a discussion of documenting change and calculating costs and utility analysis.

23. Discuss Sovie's (1985) list of strategies for managing resources more productively.

    See Box on pp. 89-90

24. Discuss methods of standardizing the nature of patient days and estimating the validity of measurements made by patient classification systems.

    a. use patient classification system calculation of required hours of care, divide by 24 hours to produce required days of care (p. 84)
    b. look for discussion of case mix and factors used to cluster patients (e.g., DRGs) (p. 80)

CHAPTER 6 - ETHICS IN HEALTH CARE

<u>TRUE/FALSE</u>

1. Two theories in biomedical ethics are deontology, which looks at the rightness or wrongness of actions based on the resulting consequences, and teleology, which focuses on the rightness or wrongness of duties and obligations.

2. The human advocacy concept proposes that the nurse provide information to the patient and family, assist in making decisions which do not conflict with the patient's value system, and help the patient find meaning and purpose in the issues they face.

3. Four principles form the foundation of biomedical ethics. These principles are: 1) autonomy, 2) nonmaleficence, 3) beneficence, and 4) justice.

4. Models to aid in ethical decision making should <u>not</u> incorporate the nursing process and the principles of biomedical ethics.

5. Crisham's model for ethical decision making, MORAL, is made up of five steps: M -massage the dilemma, O - outline options, R - review criteria and resolve, A -affirm position and act, L - look back

Answers:
>   1) False, p. 101
>   2) True, p. 102
>   3) True, pp.102-4
>   4) False, p. 104
>   5) True, pp.104-5

<u>MULTIPLE CHOICE</u>;

6. The principle of autonomy specifically refers to all of the following <u>except</u>: (p. 102)

    * a. helping the client gain what is of benefit to him/her
      b. allowing the client freedom of choice to make decisions
      c. protecting the privacy of the client in health matters
      d. providing informed consent
      e. recognizing the client's right to know and to refuse treatment

7. The principle of beneficence, specifically, implies which of the following? (p. 103)

      a. to protect the client's right to privacy
      b. to provide informed consent
    * c. to do good and avoid doing harm
      d. to give the client his or her own right or due

8. Which of the following is <u>not</u> a true statement regarding the Code of Ethics?

(pp. 99-100)

    a. It is based on beliefs about the nature of individuals, nursing, health, and society.
    b. It provides guidance for conduct and relationships in carrying out nursing responsibilities consistent with ethical obligations.
    c. It was devised by the American Nurses Association.
 * d. It gives specific answers for ethical dilemmas.

Situation 1
You are an OR surgical nurse, and a patient to whom you are assigned is scheduled to have an elective abortion in the a.m. You are opposed to this procedure on religious and moral grounds. You have thus requested to exchange cases with another surgical nurse who is scheduled to work also, but she has refused your request. To not assist may cause harm to the patient.

9.   Professional ethics dictates which of the following? (p. 103)

       a. you may refuse to assist with the procedure
 *   b. you may not refuse to assist with the procedure
       c. you may call in sick

10.   Which principle would apply to this situation? (p. 103)

       a. the principle of nonmaleficence
 *   b. the principle of beneficence
       c. the principle of justice
       d. the principle of autonomy

Situation 2

Mrs. Gentry is an 89 year old patient who was admitted with congestive heart failure. You have been her primary nurse for one week. She has expressed to you several times that she is ready to die and wants no heroic measures performed should her condition worsen. She has a sudden stroke when you are there and is comatose. Her son arrives and states to the doctor that he wants everything possible done to keep his mother alive.

11.   Your responsibility in this situation is: (pp. 102-103)

       a. to do or say nothing to the son or doctor regarding the patient's wishes
       b. to encourage the doctor to abide by the son's request
 *   c. to share Mrs. Gentry's comments with the son and the physician, hoping that the patient's desires will be considered

12.   The principle relating to this situation is which of the following? (pp. 102-103)

       a. the principle of maleficence
       b. the principle of beneficence
       c. the principle of justice

         * d. the principle of autonomy

13. The statement for the Code for Nurses: (p. 100)

        a. evaluate the quality of nursing school curricula
        b. define the scope of nursing practice in a given state
    * c. provide guidance for conduct and relationships in carrying
           outnursing responsibilities consistent with the ethical
           obligations of the profession and quality nursing care
        d. prescribe actions for specific nursing care situations

14. The ethical principle, upon which most nursing codes of ethics are based, is: (p. 103)

        a. autonomy
        b. beneficence
        c. justice
    * d. nonmaleficence

15. The term "beneficence" means: (p. 103)

        a. do no harm
        b. fairness
    * c. do good
        d. personal liberty

ESSAY QUESTIONS:

16. Why is ethics integral to nursing?

    See ANA Code for Nurses, Fig. 6-1, p. 100, Ethical dilemmas and conflicting obligations are a daily occurrence for a nurse manager.

17. Discuss the different ethical approaches or philosophies.

    deontology - universal principles that are inherently good or right, regardless of their consequences.

    teleology - the rightness or wrongness of actions is gauged by their ends or consequences. (p. 101)

18. Name and discuss the basic principles of biomedical ethics.

    autonomy - self-governance
    nonmaleficence - do no harm
    beneficence - doing good
    justice - giving each his right or due (pp. 102-4)

19. Discuss the 5-step model of ethics presented in the text.

    M=massage the dilemma

O=outline options
R=review criteria and resolve
A=affirm position and act
L=look back (pp. 104-5)

20.   Identify several special ethical issues for nurses and discuss each.

       This is an open question

21.   Discuss the use of a decision matrix such as that of Crisham presented
       in Figure 6-2 of the text for resolving ethical dilemmas.

       See Fig. 6-2, p. 107. This is an open question.

22.   Using the MORAL model of Crisham, discuss the case study of Mrs. Y
       presented in the text.

       This is an open question. See pp. 105-108

23.   List and discuss several special ethical issues faced by nurse
       managers.

       a. provision of safe care
       b. confronting unsafe practice
       c. supporting patient and staff autonomy
       d. beneficence/nonmalficence
       e. compliance with policy/M.D. orders (p. 108)

24.   Describe the ANA Code for Nurses.

       See Figure 6-1, p. 100

25.   Describe the ANA Standards of Nursing Practice (or the AHA Patient Bill
       of Rights, Canadian Nurses Association Code of Ethics, Consumer's
       Association of Canada Consumer Rights in Health Care).

CHAPTER 7 - COMMUNICATION AND INFORMATION SYSTEMS

TRUE/FALSE

1. Communication involves knowledge of management and communication theories, people and the context of organizations.

2. Studies indicate that gender impacts many aspects of communication.

3. Oral communication contains both verbal and nonverbal components.

4. The ability to listen is not an important element of effective communication.

5. The process of learning active listening skills requires paying more attention to forming a response than paying attention to another's message.

6. Aggressiveness implies behaviors that a person uses to stand up for himself and his/her rights without violating the rights of others.

7. Communication channels used by a nurse manager may be downward, upward, and diagonal.

8. There are few computerized systems that can be applied to nursing.

Answers:

1) True, p. 116	5) False, p. 125
2) True, p. 121	6) False, p. 128
3) True, p. 124	7) True, p. 132
4) False, p. 125	8) False, pp.134-151

MULTIPLE CHOICE

9. Which of the following are limitations of the Shannon-Weaver model of communication? (p. 116)

    a. focuses on the sender's ability to prepare messages and ignores inferences that the receiver makes
    b. indicates that the receiver's message follows the sender's, when in fact, communication may be occurring concurrently
    c. allows for no provisions of nonverbal communications which makes up a large portion of most exchanges
    d. a and b
  * e. all of the above

10. Various models of communication include all of the following except: (pp. 116-119)

        a. Shannon-Weaver model
        b. strategic choice model
        c. Targowski and Bowman's model
    *   d. societal-cultural listening model

11. Factors which need to be considered that influence management
    communication are all of the following except: (p. 121)

        a. gender
        b. culture
        c. organizational climate
    *   d. age

12. Which of the following is not a component of organizational culture
    that impacts communication? (p. 122)

    *   a. gender
        b. customs
        c. climate
        d. objective and subjective culture

13. Which of the following areas of nonspeech best describes nonverbal
    communication? (pp. 125-126)

        a. kinetics, or body movements and gestures
        b. spatial relationships between communicants
    *   c. written communication
        d. paralanguage or nonlanguage verbalizations that affect speech
           (pitch, tone, timing, pace, voice)
        e. cultural attributes and appearance (clothing, grooming, hair
           style)

14. One of the first applications of computers in patient care was in
    _____ (p. 135)

        a. computerized Kardexes
    *   b. patient monitoring
        c. staffing and scheduling
        d. training and evaluation

15. A Nursing Information System assists the nurse in all of the following
    ways except: (p. 147)

        a. to determine a nursing diagnosis
        b. to develop a nursing care plan

        c. to recommend interventions and determine
           evaluation strategies
        d. to determine the number of patient care hours needed
           based on patient acuity
    *   e. to analyze trends in patient responses

16. Which steps are important to remember when instituting computerization? (p. 151)

      a. define the computing needs of the unit based on goals
      b. choose the appropriate hardware and software configuration
      c. install the computer system first and worry about needs of the unit, hardware and software later
  * d. a and b
      e. c only

ESSAY QUESTIONS

17. That aspect of the human brain or mind that is responsible for the processing of communication is called the <u>Cognitive Management Apparatus</u>. Name and define the four linking processes within it. (p. 119)

  1. The <u>information-steering process</u> - the system that manages the transmission of data
  2. The <u>decision-making process</u> - the system that categorizes information and determines the importance of knowledge
  3. The <u>behavior process</u> - the system that determines what action needs to be taken in order to process the information
  4. The <u>business communication process</u> - the system that generates the messages from the sender and interprets the message from the receiver

18. List the ten different layers from which communication is sent. (p. 119-120)

  1. the physical link
  2. the systems link
  3. the audience link
  4. the session link
  5. the environment link
  6. the functions role link
  7. the symbols link
  8. the behavior link
  9. the values link
  10. the storage/retrieval link

19. List the principles that should be applied to techniques of effective communication (pp. 123-124)

  1. Information given is not communication
  2. Responsibility for clarity resides with the sender
  3. Use simple and exact language
  4. Encourage feedback
  5. The sender must have credibility
  6. Acknowledgement of others is essential
  7. Use direct channels of communication

20. Give examples or sources of distorted communication. (p. 127)

    a. The sender may write or speak without adequate reasoning.
    b. The sender may use inadequate or judgmental words.
    c. The sender may speak too fast or too slow.
    d. The receiver may be busy or distracted.
    e. The sender may use unfamiliar words to the receiver.
    f. The sender may spend so much time on detail that the receiver misses the main point.

21. Identify the Ten Basic Rights for Women in the Health Professions according to Chenevert. (pp. 128-131)

    1. You have the right to be treated with respect.
    2. You have the right to a reasonable work load.
    3. You have the right to an equitable wage.
    4. You have the right to determine your own priorities.
    5. You have the right to ask for what you want.
    6. You have the right to refuse without making excuses or feeling guilty.
    7. You have the right to make mistakes and be responsible for them.
    8. You have the right to give and receive information as a professional.
    9. You have the right to act in the best interest of the patient.
    10. You have the right to be human.

CHAPTER 8 - MOTIVATING STAFF

TRUE/FALSE

1. Motivational theories are classified into two different groups which are: content theories or process theories.

2. Process theories generally include instinct theories and need theories.

3. Expectancy theory suggests that people's thoughts about, and evaluation of, the environment and events are important determinants of behavior.

4. Job enrichment focuses on the addition of tasks in order to increase the variety of skills and talents that staff members must use in the performance of their jobs.

5. Change in any organization seldom creates resistance.

6. Punishment is more effective in changing behavior than positive reinforcement.

Answers:

1. True, p. 155	4. False, p. 173	
2. False, p. 155	5. False, p. 32	
3. True, p. 162	6. False, p. 178	

MULTIPLE CHOICE

Situation 1

The decision has been made to implement a clinical nursing ladder at a general hospital to promote retention of registered nurses. Ms. Kremer, nurse manager, has discussed with her staff rewards for staff members when agreed-upon goals are met.

7. Ms. Bennett, clinical nurse, believes that she can actually perform the requirements for advancing to the next clinical nurse level. The perception of her ability is referred to as: (p. 162)

      a. instrumentality
    * b. expectancy
      c. valence
      d. equity

8. When Ms. Bennett participates in goal setting, high performance is most likely when: (p. 168)

      a. general goals are agreed upon by the nurse and nurse manager
      b. there are specific incentives rather than goals
      c. specific goals are easily accomplished
    * d. specific, difficult goals are set

Situation 2

Ms. Marshall, nurse manager of a general medical nursing unit, has been asked to implement several changes on her nursing unit including a new method for documentation of patient care.

9.   Ms. Marshall can increase motivation and decrease resistance to change by all of the following except: (pp. 172-178)

   * a. introducing the changed documentation method as a part of the other changes planned for the nursing unit
      b. meeting with staff and discussing the reasons for using the new method
      c. planning the change strategy prior to introducing it to staff
      d. encouraging staff to participate in identifying problems with the present method

10.   During implementation of change on Ms. Marshall's nursing unit, motivation and satisfaction may be increased by: (p. 172)

      a. assigning desirable aspects of tasks to high-performing staff members
   * b. asking high-performing staff members to choose from a a list of tasks
      c. assigning undesirable tasks to individuals whose performance is poor
      d. assigning undesirable tasks to those who perform them the best

11.   The "core job dimensions" according to job redesign theory are: (p. 174)

      a. task variety, significance, identify, and autonomy
      b. task variety, importance, significance, feedback and autonomy
   * c. skill variety, task significance, task identify, feedback and autonomy
      d. task importance, interaction, task variety, autonomy, and feedback
      e. none of the above

12.   Which variable is most strongly related to performance according to goal setting theory? (p. 168)

      a. an unacceptable goal
      b. an ambiguous goal
   * c. a difficult goal
      d. an assigned goal

13.   Difficult goals lead to improved performance providing they are accepted by the: (p.168)

      a. most capable workers

        b. majority of workers
    * c. individual
        d. organization

14.   Which of the needs in Maslow's hierarchy has the highest priority
       (comes first)? (p. 156)

           a. belongingness and love (identification, affection)
           b. safety (security, health)
           c. self-actualization (self-fulfillment, personal growth)
        * d. physiological (hunger, thirst, etc.)

15.   Which theory proposes that an individual sets up a ratio of his inputs
       to his outcomes and compares the value of that ratio with the ratio for
       a relevant comparison person? (p. 165)

           a. hierarchy theory
           b. drive theory
           c. VIE theory
        * d. Adams' Equity theory

16.   The two major components of Vroom's theory of motivation are: (p. 162)

           a. drive, reward
        * b. instrumentality, expectancy
           c. considerate, initiating structure
           d. satisfiers, dissatisfiers

17.   It has as its objective explaining why people behave as they do.
       (p. 157)

        * a. a process theory
           b. need hierarchy
           c. balance theory
           d. work theory
           e. board class processes

18.   In Vroom's theory of motivation, <u>instrumentality</u> is defined as:
       (p. 162)

           a. the effective orientation of individuals toward
               particular outcomes
        * b. the degree to which a person sees an action as leading
               to a desired outcome
           c. the degree to which a person sees certain outcomes as probable
           d. none of these

19.   John is always late to work. His supervisor yells at him every day.
       John comes into work on time. There is no yelling. John then
       continues to come into work on time. This is an example of
       (p. 158-159)

a. positive reinforcement
* b. negative reinforcement
c. punishment
d. none of the above

ESSAY QUESTIONS:

20. From a managerial perspective, do you think the content approach or the process approach to motivation is the most useful?

Student opinion will differ substantially; however, often most students vote for process theory, especially goal setting, because it is a specific technique that managers can implement with employees. Expectancy theory is also an applied theory in a more general sense. (pp. 155, 162)

21. What implications does Maslow's need hierarchy have for the design of organizational reward systems? Is it easier or harder to design rewards for individuals operating at upper levels of the hierarchy rather than at lower levels?

The need hierarchy suggests that individuals have different needs because they are at different levels of hierarchy. Thus, a reward system should be developed considering the need level that is active with specific employees. For example, for upper-level managers, esteem and self-actualization needs are probably very important. Without question, designing rewards that satisfy upper-level needs is a more difficult task. To illustrate this point, ask students to consider the difficulty of designing rewards that fulfill self-actualization needs compared to designing rewards that satisfy physiological needs. (p. 156)

22. Many factors other than motivation influence productivity. What are some of these other factors and how can a manager know which factors, including motivation, to focus on to improve productivity? (This chapter and the Productivity Chapter)

One reason why productivity improvement programs are so challenging for management is because of the many factors involved. Besides employee motivation, productivity is affected by the quality of the equipment used by the employee, the employee's ability, job experience and problem-solving skills. Effective leadership significantly influences productivity and so does the reward system. A manager can determine the factors that require attention by evaluating the factors before implementing a productivity improvement program. (p. 24-37)

23. Do you think organizations want all employees to be self-actualized? What sort of problems would managers face in that sort of organization?

Few organizations want such a situation because the organization

95

would be faced with the insurmountable task of providing satisfying jobs and rewards for these employees. (p. 156)

24. Define process theory. How do process theories differ from content theories? (pp. 155-169)

    a. Process theories help explain and predict what initiates, sustains, and terminates behavior while content theories only help us understand what outcomes people desire to attain.
    b. Process theories can be used to predict and attempt to control. Content theories are usually only useful for understanding.

25. What is job design? What is the difference between job enlargement and job enrichment? What are the components of Hackman and Oldham's model? Using a specific nursing unit, (e.g., intensive care, psychiatry) apply the Hackman and Oldham model.

    Job design is the process for designing or deciding which tasks are done in a position or job. Job enlargement is adding more tasks at the same level while job enrichment is adding more tasks across different levels.

    See p. 175, Figure 8-3 for the model.

26. Describe the integrated model of motivation presented in Chapter 9 of your text.

    See Figure 8-2, p. 171

CHAPTER 9 - LEADERSHIP SKILLS

TRUE/FALSE

1. The term leadership is synonymous with the term management.

2. Management is the use of one's skills to influence others to perform to the best of their ability.

3. Referent power is based upon admiration and respect for an individual as a person.

4. The Pygmalion effect (or self-fulfilling prophecy) refers to a situation where what is envisioned about a person or situation becomes what is expected.

5. Research shows that most managers have difficulty building an effective team.

6. Cohesiveness is an unimportant element in effecting performance of a team.

Answers:

1.	False, p. 181	4.	True, p. 193
2.	False, p. 181	5.	True, p. 195
3.	True, p. 182	6.	False, p. 195

MULTIPLE CHOICE:

7. Leadership is best described as: (p. 181)

    * a. an interpersonal relationship in which the leader employs specific behaviors and strategies to influence individuals and groups toward goal setting and attainment
    b. the coordination and integration of resources through planning, organizing, directing and controlling in order to accomplish specific instructional goals and objectives.
    c. the coordination of the basic work activities of an organizational unit in accordance with plans and procedures.

8. Leadership implies: (p. 181)

    a. domination
    b. getting work done through other people
    c. making people want to accomplish something
    d. a & b
    * e. b & c

9. Leadership is _informal_ when: (p. 182)

    a. practiced by the designated nurse in charge of the unit

    * b. practiced by a team member who is not designated as the nurse in

charge

10. A leader has power to the extent that: (p. 182)

   a. the group members think the leader controls and will use rewards as punishment to back up requests
   b. the group members either greatly fear or value highly the outcomes that may result
   c. the group members have few alternatives
   d. b and c only
 * e. all of the above

11. A nurse manager who is experienced and knowledgeable regarding leadership is said to possess which kind of power? (p. 182)

   a. coercive power
   b. reward power
   c. referent power
 * d. expert power

12. Referent power is based upon: (p. 182)

   a. particular knowledge and skill not possessed by group members
 * b. admiration and respect for an individual as a person
   c. the negative things a leader might do to individuals or group members

13. Authoritarian leadership styles are: (p. 185)

   a. primarily concerned with human relations and teamwork
 * b. primarily concerned with task accomplishment rather than relationships
   c. tend to have few established goals or policies

14. Effective leadership is a joint function of leader characteristics and situational characteristics. This is the general theme of: (p. 186)

   a. the Path Goal theory
 * b. Fiedler's Contingency Model
   c. Social Learning theory

15. Of the three major determinants of the leadership situation, which is the most important according to Fiedler? (p. 187)

 * a. leader-member relations
   b. task structure
   c. position power
   d. all are equally important

16. In Fiedler's contingency theory of leadership, the effectiveness of a leader depends upon a match between: (p. 186)

        a. bass centered behavior and subordinate centered behavior
        b. task motivated behavior and relationship motivated behavior
    *   c. the leadership style and the situation requirements

17. Which school of leadership utilized the terms "consideration" and
     "initiating structure" as descriptors of leader behaviors? (p. 183)

        a. Bales - Harvard
    *   b. Stagdill - Ohio State
        c. Fiedler - Illinois
        d. Katz and Kahn - Michigan

18. The path-goal approach to leadership has its theoretical assumptions
     based on which theory of motivation? (p. 188)

        a. equity theory
        b. operant conditioning
        c. need theory
    *   d. expectancy theory

19. Which of the following types of leader behavior would be most effective
     when subordinates view their job as boring, frustrating, stressful or
     unpleasant? (p. 188)

        a. directive leadership behavior
        b. achievement oriented behavior
    *   c. supportive leadership behavior
        d. participative leadership behavior

20. The Pygmalion effect is best described as: (p. 193)

        a. behaviors that although learned, cannot be effectively performed
            without practice
    *   b. the self-fulfilling prophecy in which an individual or situation
            becomes what one expects it to be
        c. the use of one's skills to influence others to perform to the
            best of their ability

ESSAY QUESTIONS:

21. Define and discuss the bases of power as presented in the text.
     (p. 182-183)

            reward power
            punishment (coercive power)
            information power
            legitimate power
            expert power
            referent power

22. Define leadership and how it differs from management.

See page 181

23. What are the three questions you should ask yourself before implementing a particular leadership style according to Vroom and his leadership style flow chart? (p. 91)

    1. Do I have all of the information needed to make the decision?
    2. Is acceptance by subordinates required for effective implementation?
    3. If I delegate, will subordinates make a decision I can live with?

24. Identify several theories of leadership. What are the major propositions of each? How does one differ from the other?

    This is an open question depending upon the theories chosen for discussion. See pp. 186-193 for the theories

25. Define and describe social learning theory. Why should the nurse manager be concerned with role modeling? Describe an incident where you learned through the use of a role model. (p. 192-193)

    Social learning theory recognizes that individuals not only learn by education, but by observing role models, seeing role models positively reinforced for modeling correct behaviors and by practicing key behaviors. Therefore, staff nurses can learn from the nurse manager's expert role modeling.

26. Describe various factors which affect group cohesiveness. (p. 195-196)

    a. physical proximity of group members
    b. frequency of interaction and the expectation of future interaction
    c. management of the communication processes
    d. structure of the task
    e. common group goal
    f. characteristics of group members

CHAPTER 10 - STRESS AND TIME MANAGEMENT

TRUE/FALSE

1. Stress is the individual's reaction to internal and/or external demands which pose a threat.

2. Stress is the body's response to negative occurrences; it is not present when the occurrences are positive.

3. Stress may come from many different areas such as job tasks, the physical environment, the supervisor's behavior, institutional factors, changing environmental, societal or nursing traditions.

4. Undue, prolonged anxiety, depression, sudden changes in mood and behavior, perfectionism and physical illnesses are all warning signs of too much stress.

5. People can pursue productive lives without resolving the stress in their lives.

6. It is important that the nurse manager learn to use time well. The setting of priorities can be beneficial to accomplishing this goal.

7. Delegation can play an important role in utilizing time well. By delegating, the nurse manager can reduce personal time demands.

8. When delegating, the nurse manager should follow a series of steps to ensure success. These steps include: planning before delegating, defining the responsibility in terms of specific results to be achieved, determining the authority and limits to be delegated, not taking over for the subordinate, not holding the subordinate accountable, selecting the subordinate carefully and making effective assignments.

9. While some responsibilities may be effectively delegated, others cannot. The nurse manager should not delegate in any of the following areas: disciplining an immediate subordinate, unit morale problems or areas where the nurse manager has legal acountability.

10. The nurse manager should strive to have an "open communication" policy where time will be made to discuss something which is really important rather than an "open door" policy where anyone can telephone or drop in at any time.

Answers:
1.	True,	p. 201	6.	True, p. 215
2.	False,	p. 201	7.	True, p. 215
3.	True,	pp. 201-204	8.	False, pp. 216-218
4.	True,	p. 207	9.	True, p. 217
5.	False,	p. 208	10.	False, p. 210

MULTIPLE CHOICE:

11.   Which of the following statements is not true regarding stress?
        (p. 201)

                a. Stress is the reaction of individuals to demands from the
                    enviornment that pose a threat.
                b. The body's response to the conflict caused by two or more
                    incompatible demands results in stress.
                c. The response to stress is the same whether the stressor is
                    positive or negative.
            *   d. All stress should be absent in order to sustain life.

12.   Which of the following can be categorized as antecedents to stress?
        (p. 203)

            *   a. organizational, interpersonal and individual factors
                b. depression and prolonged anxiety
                c. negative coping behaviors

13.   Which of the following is not an organizational antecedent to stress?
        (pp. 203-204)

                a. job task overload
                b. insufficient information on assignment
                c. authoritarian supervisory behavior
            *   d. multiple roles of spouse, parent, nurse
                e. rapidly changing health environment

Situation 1

You are a nurse manager on a busy open heart unit. Recently you are feeling
increasingly stressed and burned out. You have begun to experience physical
symptoms of hypertension, migraine headaches, and colitis. You have
identified the major stressors in your life as organizational factors. You
wish to begin a stress management regime.

14.   Which of the following interventions would be helpful in managing your
        stress? (p. 208)

                a. identify and accept your limitations
                b. develop outside interests
                c. exercise regularly
                d. learn how to relax
            *   e. all of the above

15.   You are attempting to utilize more positive coping responses. Which of
        the following is not an appropriate positive coping response? (p. 208)

                a. redefine and clarify your roles
                b. practice effective time management
            *   c. call in sick when you feel stressed

102

Situation 2

Not only are you experiencing stress as a nurse manager, but you have noticed
that many of the staff on your unit are frequently calling in sick, resigning,
and showing signs of decreased productivity. You are truly concerned about
their welfare as well as that of the patients and institution. You want to
assist them in dealing with their stress.

16.   Your first priority in attempting to deal with their stressors is to:
        (p. 208)

            *   a. identify the source of stress
                b. decide how you can eliminate the stress
                c. give each one a personal day off
                d. clarify their roles and activities

17.   You have notified higher administration and asked their assistance in
        helping to decrease the stress of your workers. In which of the
        following ways could higher administration be most helpful? (p. 210)

                a. allow greater participation in decision making
                b. encourage a network of social support
                c. keep communication channels open
                d. increase skills training even for experienced staff
            *   e. all of the above

Situation 3

Ms. Kiely is a manager of a neuro intensive care unit which employs a large
staff of nurses. There is no assistant head nurse so Ms. Kiely is responsible
for all management functions for the unit. She rarely delegates activities to
the other staff. Ms. Kiely often takes work home with her and is slowly
experiencing burnout as a result of feeling tired and overworked. She has
vowed to begin to establish a time management regime.

18.   To be an effective delegator, one must have a thorough understanding
        and use of which of the following concepts? (p. 216)

                a. power and influence
                b. autonomy and control
                c. coercive and reward power
            *   d. the granting of authority

19.   The key steps in delegation do not include: (p. 216)

                a. responsibility
                b. authority
                c. accountability

            *   d. controlling
                e. all of the above

20. Which of the following statements is <u>not</u> true in describing authority? (p. 216)

      a. it is closely associated with legitimate power
      b. it can and should be shared with subordinates
      c. it resides in the position, not the person
   * d. it is synonymous with responsibility

21. Ms. Kiely has attempted to identify some of the reasons why she feels uncomfortable delegating responsibilities to her staff. Which of the following could be possible obstacles to delegation? (p. 217)

      a. fear of losing control
      b. failure to set goals and timetables
      c. lack of subordinates' abilities
      d. fear of subordinate incompetence
   * e. all of the above

22. Which area of responsibility could Ms. Kiely appropriately learn to delegate to another staff nurse? (p. 217)

      a. disciplining an immediate subordinate
      b. handling morale problems on the unit
      c. termination of another staff nurse
   * d. checking and ordering supplies for the unit

<u>Situation 4</u>

Ms. Kiely has great difficulty in managing her time efficiently. She allows numerous interruptions such as telephone calls and drop-in visitors and has difficulty setting priorities. She has set a goal to work on these areas.

23. Which of the following telephone responses can assist in minimizing small talk and socializing? (p. 219)

   * a. "Hello...what can I do for you?"
      b. "Hello...what are you doing today?"
      c. "Hello...how are you?"

24. Ms. Kiely has numerous visitors each day who demand much of her time. Which of the following suggestions would be <u>least</u> effective in handling visitors? (p. 220)

      a. meet visitors outside the office
      b. use stand-up conversations when a drop-in-visitor appears
      c. encourage appointments when possible
   * d. arrange desk so that she can be seen by passerby
      e. keep staff informed by memos or routing slips

ESSAY QUESTIONS

25.   Discuss role ambiguity and role conflict

        See definitions, p. 205

26.   Other than for humanitarian reasons, why should organizations be
        concerned about the physical and mental health consequences of work
        stress?

        Organizations should be concerned because a growing number of
        employees are suing their employers to obtain compensation for
        illnesses allegedly caused by excessive job stress. These
        employees consider their employers liable for the costs (financial
        and psychological) of their illnesses. Although the interpretation
        of the law on this issue is still evolving in the courts and
        employers are winning most of the cases, some employees have won
        major awards. Stress management will also lower absenteeism,
        turnover, and use of sick leave. (see entire chapter)

27.   Of the individual approaches to managing stress discussed in this
        chapter, which one appeals to you the most? Which one the least?
        Explain.

        This is an open question. See list p. 208

28.   What is the relationship between work stress and work motivation? If
        we could eliminate all stress, what effect would this have on
        motivation? Explain.

        Stress at work can motivate up to a certain point. Many have found
        that such stress sharpens the senses, and increases adrenalin and
        involvement in a somewhat stressful task. However, if the stress
        level exceeds the individual's optimal stress point (see Figure 11-
        1), stress diminishes motivation and performance. The individual
        feels overloaded by stress, and efforts to cope with the stressors
        leave little energy to muster the motivation to focus on a task and
        perform well. Too little or no stress at all is also de-
        motivating.

29.   Discuss strategies that managers and institutions can use to lessen
        employee stress.

        See pp. 208-210

30.   Discuss the Stress Diagnostic Survey (or the Social Readjustment Rating
        Scale).

        Use this question only if you have the students fill out these
        instruments. (See Figure 10-3, p. 206; 10-4, p. 209)

31.   When is time wasted? What are the major types of time wasters? How
        may each of these be decreased? Identify the major wasters of your

time. Time is wasted when it is devoted to something other than what really needs to be done. The major types of time wasters are interruptions, telephone calls, paging and beeping, drop-in visitors and paperwork. (pp. 211-212)

Delegation can be used to help in time management. Delegation means sharing responsibility and authority with subordinates and holding them accountable for performance. The benefits of delegation include more time for high priority objectives, developing staff potential, identifying strengths and weaknesses of staff, and fostering a team relationship. The three important concepts are responsibility, authority and accountability. (p. 216)

32. What two decisions must be made when delegating authority? What steps can be taken to assure effective delegation of authority? What should never be delegated? Why? (See pp. 216-217)

33. Describe and discuss an interruption log. (See p. 219)

34. Describe methods to manage time spent on the phone.

    a. plan calls
    b. minimize small talk and socializing
    c. set a time aside each day for calls
    d. use a timer
    e. state and ask for preferred times (pp. 219-220)

35. Describe methods to manage drop-in visitors.

    a. meet visitors outside of office
    b. keep visits short
    c. stay in control
    d. encourage appointments
    e. keep staff informed
    f. arrange furniture to discourage conversation
    g. go to see others (p. 220)

36. Identify the paper work associated with the nurse manager's job. What methods might be used so that this work is completed more effectively?

    This is an open question; see pp. 221-222

CHAPTER 11 - CRITICAL THINKING

TRUE/FALSE

1. Problem solving is a higher level cognitive process which includes critical thinking and decision making.

2. Problem solving and decision making are synonymous.

3. Experimentation is a type of problem solving.

4. Satisficing is a decision making strategy.

5. The key element in decision making under conditions of risk is to accurately determine the probabilities of each alternative.

6. Brainstorming and synectics are useful techniques in promoting creativity.

7. Decisions may be made under conditions of certainty, risk and uncertainty.

Answers:

1.	False, p. 227	5.	True, p. 234
2.	False, p. 227	6.	True, p. 245
3.	True, p. 228	7.	True, p. 233
4.	True, p. 233		

MULTIPLE CHOICE:

8.   Critical thinking can best be described as: (p. 226)

 * a. a higher level cognitive process which includes problem solving and decision making
   b. a subset of problem solving
   c. a process that is used when a gap is perceived between some existing state and some desired state

9.   Which of the following methods are sometimes used to solve problems? (p. 228-229)

   a. trial and error
   b. experimentation
   c. past experience
 * d. all of the above
   e. a and c

10.   The most important part of problem solving is to: (p. 230)

 * a. define the problem
   b. gather information
   c. analyze the information

d. develop solutions
e. make a decision

11. Decision making can best be defined as: (p. 233)

    a. a higher level cognitive process which includes creative problem solving
  * b. the process of establishing criteria by which alternative courses of action are developed and selected
    c. a process used when a gap is perceived between an existing state and a desired state

12. Which of the following are decision-making strategies? (p. 233)

    a. satisficing
    b. optimizing
    c. risk
  * d. a and b
    e. c only

13. Within an organization, nurse managers make decisions under which of the following conditions? (p. 233)

  * a. certainty, risk or uncertainty
    b. optimizing or satisficing
    c. maximax approach or maximin approach

14. The most common decision-making condition is that of: (p. 234)

    a. certainty
  * b. risk
    c. uncertainty

15. Which of the following approaches to decision making would the nurse manager most likely use in situations of uncertainty? (p. 235)

    a. the maximax approach
    b. the maximin approach
    c. the risk averting approach
  * d. all of the above
    e. a and b

16. The maximin approach of decision making is best described as: (p. 235)

    a. selecting an alternative whose best possible outcome is the best possible outcome for all alternatives.
  * b. to compare the worst possible outcomes for each of the possible alternatives and choose the one that seems the least objectionable
    c. choose the alternative with the least variation among its possible outcomes

17.   Creativity is best described as: (p. 243)

      a. the use of one's brain to "storm" a creative problem in a group meeting in rapid fashion
* b. the ability to develop new and better solutions
      c. the process of problem solving

18.   Which of the following is not characteristic of a creative person according to Steiner? (p. 244)

* a. prefers simple and easily understood thought processes to complex ones
      b. generates ideas rapidly
      c. has a tendency to provide original solutions to problems
      d. views authority as conventional rather than absolute

19.   Synectics, a method for stimulating creativity, is best described as: (p. 245)

* a. concentrates on generating a large number of ideas
      b. concentrates on trying to identify one new idea
      c. asks group members to identify with the problems
      d. attempts to describe the problem using impersonal images

ESSAY QUESTIONS:

20.   How can a nurse manager develop the critical thinking process? What series of questions would be asked when examining a specific problem or making a decision? (p. 227)

      a. What are the underlying assumptions?
      b. How was evidence interpreted?
      c. How are the arguments to be evaluated?

21.   Differentiate between problem solving and decision making. (p. 227)

Problem solving involves diagnosing a problem and solving it. This may or may not entail deciding on the one correct solution. Decision making may or may not involve a problem, but it always involves selecting an alternative from several, each of which could be appropriate under certain circumstances.

22.   List the seven steps of the problem solving process. (p. 229)

      a. define the problem
      b. gather information
      c. analyze the information
      d. develop solutions
      e. make a decision
      f. implement the decision
      g. evaluate the solution

23.   List the seven step decision making process. (pp. 237-242)

        a. identify the purpose
        b. set criteria
        c. weigh the criteria
        d. seek alternatives
        e. test alternatives
        f. troubleshoot
        g. evaluate the action

24.   List and describe various stumbling blocks to problem solving and decision making experienced by nurse managers. (p. 242-243)

        a. personality traits
        b. inexperience
        c. lack of adaptability
        d. preconceived ideas

25.   Describe the four stages of creativity according to Wallas. (p. 243)

        a. preparation
        b. incubation
        c. insight (illumination)
        d. verification

26.   Describe characteristics of a creative person.

        See list on page 244

27.   List the four basic rules that must be understood and followed in order to obtain maximum creativity from a group using the brain storming technique.

        See list on page 245

28.   How can a nurse manager help stimulate the generation of new ideas from his/her group? (pp. 246-247)

        1. Design a carefully planned program
        2. Meet with new employees routinely as part of the orientation process to seek information about problems
        3. Foster creativity by establishing ground rules that permit innovative managers and staff to function without fear of reprisals or termination if they fail. Reward creativity.
        4. Create a climate for the survival of potentially useful ideas. Build an attitude favorable to giving new ideas a fair and proper hearing. Reduce the tendency to destroy the creative process within individuals and groups. Encourage creative change of ideas among other units.

CHAPTER 12 - MANAGING GROUPS

TRUE/FALSE

1. Informal groups are a part of the organizational design and may be temporary or permanent.

2. A group is composed of individuals usually sharing differentiated roles to achieve common goals.

3. An important function of the nurse manager role is facilitating problem solving and communication with different levels in the organization.

4. Norms are formal rules of behavior which are specific to a group member's position in the group.

5. When group cohesiveness is low, employee productivity can be expected to vary widely.

Answers:

1. False, Chapter 12, p. 250
2. True   p. 250
3. True   p. 250
4. False   p. 253
5. False   p. 254

MULTIPLE CHOICE:

6. A group is a collection of individuals who have: (p. 250)

        a. dissimilar norms
        b. identical roles
    *   c. common goals
        d. homogeneous needs

7. All of the following are examples of <u>formal</u> groups <u>except</u>: (p. 250)

        a. command groups
        b. task groups
    *   c. special interest groups
        d. task forces and committees

8. A group that includes a nurse, physician, dietitian and social worker for the purpose of planning patient care is an example of: (p. 250)

        a. a command group
    *   b. a task group
        c. a task force
        d. an informal group

9. The formal diagonal group is composed of members from: (p. 250)

        a. the same work group
        b. different organizational levels
    *   c. different departments
        d. the same nursing unit

10. According to Homans' model, the emergent group system is affected by all of the following background factors <u>except</u>: (p. 251)

        a. personal characteristics
        b. external status
        c. organizational requirements
    *   d. group roles

11. Which of the following is not an essential element of Homans' framework? (p. 251)

        a. activities
    *   b. external status
        c. interactions
        d. attitudes

12. In the process of group development, <u>storming</u> occurs when the group members: (p. 251)

        a. come together
    *   b. compete for power and status
        c. accept goals
        d. adopt rules

13. Group members begin to develop an understanding of group membership during the phase of: (p. 251)

    *   a. forming
        b. storming
        c. norming
        d. performing

14. Group members may promote group norms by all of the following activities <u>except</u>:   (p. 253)

        a. using rational argument
    *   b. minimizing the importance of the group to dissenting member
        c. using verbal attack
        d. ignoring the deviant member

15. The set of expected behaviors that define an individual's position in the group is: (p. 253)

        a. status
        b. norm
        c. leadership
    *   d. role

16. Members which tend to comply with group norms are: (p. 253)

    * a. regular members
      b. deviant members
      c. isolate members
      d. social members

17. Which of the following promote status within a group? (p. 253)

      a. not conforming to group norms
      b. dissimilar backgrounds of group members
      c. status incongruence
    * d. ability to control rewards

18. The gate-keeping function of the leadership role includes all except:
    (p. 254)

    * a. limiting communication
      b. facilitating member participation
      c. suggesting discussion procedures
      d. encouraging member suggestions

19. Uniform productivity can be expected among group members when: (p. 254)

      a. weak norms exist
      b. there is minimal cohesiveness
    * c. members enjoy participation
      d. heterogeneous attitudes are present

20. The nurse manager will find it most difficult to influence
    staff nurses when they are of: (p. 263)

    * a. common educational backgrounds
      b. varying ages
      c. different sexes
      d. dissimilar social classes

21. Individuals may join groups for which of the following reasons: (p. 256)

      a. security
      b. social support
      c. pursuit of valued goals
    * d. all of the above

22. Which of the following describes social loafing? (p. 258)

    * a. the group member produces less than expected
      b. the member receives full membership benefits
      c. it is likely to occur in very small groups
      d. it involves all group members

23. Dialectical inquiry: (p. 259)

    * a. permits disagreement through formal debate
      b. discourages alternative solutions
      c. increases the emotional aspects of conflict
      d. minimizes false assumptions

24. An advantage of group over individual decision making is that group decision making may: (p. 257)

      a. increase conflict among group members
      b. decrease time requirements
      c. decrease need for resources
    * d. increase productivity

25. Which of the following is true regarding groupthink? (p. 258)

      a. it is a positive phenomenon
      b. group members have different viewpoints
      c. it occurs when outside pressures threaten the group
    * d. the group believes it is morally right

26. The most detrimental effect of groupthink is that: (p. 258)

      a. there is no pressure for members to conform
      b. the group utilizes negative feedback
      c. members consider the ethical consequences of decisions
    * d. group decision making is ineffective

27. Reasons for the nurse manager's decision to use groups for decision making would include all of the following except: (p. 260)

    * a. no need for acceptance of the decision
      b. adequate time for decision making
      c. shared organizational goals by group members
      d. staff capability for decision making

28. Groups with more than 5 to 7 members are associated with: (p. 258)

      a. high satisfaction
      b. low absenteeism
      c. low turnover
    * d. less contribution by each team member

ESSAY QUESTIONS:

29. Discuss the conditions that contribute to groupthink.
    See p. 258

30. Describe the different types of decision making groups.
    (pp. 260-262)

ordinary interacting groups
nominal group technique
brainstorming groups
statistical aggregation
The Delphi Technique
quality circles

31. What conditions are necessary to develop effective teams?
    See 4 steps listed, p. 263

32. In order to build an effective team, what factors needs to be analyzed
    when diagnosing team problems? See questions to be asked, p. 265

33. Summarize the characteristics of an effective team.
    See team characteristics, pp. 265-266

34. Compare the similarities and differences of formal committees and
    task forces. (p. 266)

35. Describe the general guidelines for effectively leading and conducting a
    meeting. (pp. 266-269)

CHAPTER 13 - RECRUITING AND SELECTING STAFF

TRUE/FALSE

1. Job analysis is the process of determining a) the duties and responsibilities of a job, b) the tasks which must be done each day, and c) the skills, abilities, knowledge and traits needed for the job.

2. Evidence shows that applicants recruited by formal means (advertisements and employment agencies) tend to remain in a position longer than applicants recruited by informal means (recommendations by friends, rehires and walk-ins).

3. The purpose of the interview is to give and receive information as well as create a climate of good-will toward the institution offering the position.

4. Equal employment opportunity law has had two major effects on the employee selection process: tests are used more to determine the appropriateness of a potential employee and the interview process is deemphasized.

5. Selection systems must be job-related; this will eliminate problems of discrimination on the basis of race, color, sex, religion or national origin as specified by the 1964 Civil Rights Act.

Answers:

        1.   True,   p.   279
        2.   False, p.   284
        3.   True,   pp. 285-286
        4.   False, pp. 300-302
        5.   True,   pp. 300-302

MULTIPLE CHOICE:

Situation 1

A large 500 bed hospital located in the midwest is continuously involved in recruiting and selecting staff. The personnel department is initially responsible for screening and monitoring hiring practices, but the first-line managers are responsible for the final decision to hire a specific applicant. There are many processes and activities involved in the selection of a new employee.

6. Before any recruitment or selection of a new staff member is attempted, those who are responsible for hiring must <u>first</u> become familiar with which of the following? (p. 279)

    a. the past work experience of the applicant
    b. the educational level of the applicant
  * c. the job description, skills and knowledge required to perform the job

116

7. A research process that determines the duties and responsibilities of a specific job is referred to as: (p. 279)

      a. job description
      b. job specification
*   c. job analysis
      d. job knowledge

8. Which of the following techniques are available for performing job analysis? (pp. 279-282)

      a. supervisory conferences
      b. critical incidents
      c. work sampling and observation
      d. interviewing and questionnaires
*   e. all of the above
      f. none of the above

Situation 2

You are interested in applying for a job in a staff nurse position on a medical-surgical unit. You have sent in your application and have been called for an interview. You will first be screened by the personnel department and then have a face-to-face interview with the prospective head nurse.

9. To plan for the interview session as an applicant you would need to be prepared to answer questions related to which of the following areas of interest? (p. 300)

*   a. education and job history
      b. religious denomination and beliefs
      c. questions about your national origin
      d. your race

10. In order to effectively plan for the interview session, the nurse manager's primary responsibility is to: (p. 287-289)

      a. order refreshments to be served
      b. make the setting as formal as possible
*   c. review the application or resume just prior to the interview session

11. When making a decision to hire the applicant, the first step the nurse manager should consider in order of priority is: (p. 295)

*   a. weigh the qualities desired on the basis of the reliability of the data

      b. compare data across individuals in making a decision
      c. weigh the qualities required for the job in order of importance

12. The validity of the employment interview might be improved by: (pp. 295-296)

a. reaching a hiring decision early in the interview
b. contrasting each applicant to preceding applicants
c. using inexperienced interviewers
* d. none of the above

13. The assumption that an applicant's past attitudes and behavior will be predictive of job success underlies usage of which of the following selection techniques? (p. 296)

a. job knowledge tests
b. training and experience requirements
c. reference checks
* d. all of the above

14. Which of the following statements is/are true about the use of interviews in the selection process? (pp. 295-296)

a. interviews are free from the same legal requirements as tests
b. interviews tend to be very good predictors of job success
* c. interviews tend to be unreliable due to rater errors and biases
d. interviews tend to be highly job related
e. both a and c

15. Several employees wanted to be promoted to a managerial position. They were asked to perform in-basket exercises and were evaluated by trained observers. Three were selected as candidates for the job. This is an example of which of the following? (p. 300)

a. an aptitude test
* b. an assessment center
c. a performance test
d. a process of elimination
e. a confrontation technique

16. One hospital advertises job vacancies by putting a notice on bulletin boards throughout the institution. The notice contains either a summary or a complete job description, and those interested are informed about how to apply for the job. This method of recruitment is known as: (p. 284)

a. job bank
* b. job posting
c. employee referral
d. institution newsletter
e. walk-in

17. Which of the following are problems associated with observation of the job occupant as a method of job analysis? (p. 280)

a. assumes that the act of observing an individual at work does not have an impact on the work behavior itself
b. comes almost meaningless in work that is primarily mental in nature

c. not very practical when the job cycle (time from the beginning to the end of a specific task) extends over a considerable period of time
* d. all of the above are problems associated with observation of the job occupant as a method of job analysis

18. The extent to which an interview will yield similar results when administered by several interviewers is known as: (p. 295)

    a. validity
  * b. reliability
    c. probable error
    d. correlation coefficient

19. The best sources of referral (lowest turnover) are: (pp. 279-281)

    a. employee referrals
    b. newspaper ads
    c. employment agencies
    d. walk-ins and rehires
    e. both a and b
  * f. both a and d

20. Recruiting strategy is dependent upon: (p. 283)

    a. organizational image
    b. labor market conditions
    c. type of skills needed
    d. affirmative action programs
    e. a, b, and d are correct
  * f. all of the above

21. With regard to Title VII of the Civil Rights Act (as amended): (pp. 296-298)

    a. the act permits discrimination on the basis of raceor color if it can be shown that these characteristics are desired occupational qualifications
    b. the act forbids the use of professionally developedability tests
  * c. the act permits differential treatment of employees under bona fide seniority and merit systems as long as the systems were not designed with the intent to discriminate
    d. the act requires organizations to develop and implement affirmative action programs

ESSAY QUESTIONS:

22. What information should be collected in a job analysis? Why? (See p. 279)

23. What complicating factors should be anticipated in preparing to do a job analysis? (p. 279)

Not covered in text; people don't know what they are supposed to do; they will not be truthful because they hear reduction or job redesign; lack of interviewing skill on the part of the job analyst; time it will take to do.

24. Discuss the purpose of job analysis. Identify the various job analysis techniques. Discuss the pros and cons of each technique as used within nursing. (p. 279)

    a. to collect job information in order to write job descriptions design selection instruments, etc.
    b. supervisory conferences
       critical incidents
       work sampling
       observation
       interviewing
       questionnaires
       check lists

25. What are the legal issues of selection?
Compliance with EEO law and affirmative action. (pp. 295-299)

26. Identify the various selection tools. How may these be used in the selection of nurses? (entire chapter)

    a. paper and pencil tests
       work sample tests
       interviewing
       assessment centers
       references
       applications/resumes
       medical exams
    b. open question; they all can be used – see chapter

27. What steps should be followed when making the decision to hire?
(See Figure 13-1, p. 278)

28. What are the objectives of the employment interviewer? What are the principles for an effective employment interview? Discuss the development and use of the structured interview guide within nursing. Discuss the interviewing process and identify the major steps. (pp. 285-289)

    a. to gain all the job-related information possible from the candidate and give necessary information (p. 305)
    b. plan the interview
       respond to the applicant
       elicit information
       give information
       process information
    c. A Structured interview guide improves reliability, validity, guides the interview and fosters note-taking

29. What are the elements of a recruiting strategy? How do each of these elements relate to the health care industry? Discuss the impact of communication on the recruitment process. (pp. 283-285)

   a. where to look
      how to look
      when to look
      how to sell the organization
   b. See p. 13:1
   c. it is mostly done with communication media, it is the foundation of recruiting

30. What is reliability? What is validity? (pp. 295-296, 302-304)

   Reliability is a measure of the consistency of measurement. Validity is a measure of the extent to which a measurement instrument measures what it was designed to measure.

31. Describe a structured interview guide for nurses.
    (See Figure 13-5)

32. What preemployment questions are inappropriate to ask?
    (See Figure 13-8, p. 297)

33. List the key behaviors of an effective interview.
    (p. 295)

34. Describe the assessment center process.
    (See p. 298)

CHAPTER 14 – STAFF DEVELOPMENT AND PATIENT EDUCATION

TRUE/FALSE:

1. In a hospital setting, training cannot be viewed as an end in itself. Hospitals should only commit funds for training if they can reasonably expect organizational goals, such as improved patient care, lower operating costs, more efficient or better satisfied personnel, to be achieved.

2. The transfer of training from the classroom to the work place is the ultimate goal of any training program. This can best be achieved when: 1) training is as much like the job as possible, 2) training content becomes part of long-term memory, 3) training content is broken down into major steps, and 4) general principles are understood.

3. The education of adults differs from the education of children in four important areas. Adults see themselves as independent persons; they have experience which children do not have; they determine areas of information they will learn; they learn for present utilization rather than future use.

4. Evaluation is a necessary part of training, although many times it is omitted from the process or confined to those organizations who are truly committed to training.

5. Patient education has become less important in recent years because hospital stays tend to be shorter.

Answers:

    1. True,   p. 308
    2. True,   p. 311
    3. True,   p. 316
    4. True,   p. 327
    5. False, p. 327

MULTIPLE CHOICE:

Situation 1

Ms. Young is the obstetrical clinical specialist. She is in charge of OB staff development and OB patient education at a large urban hospital. She is responsible for training all OB nursing staff and assistants as well as for educating mothers regarding postnatal care of their infants before discharge. Thus, most of the staff and clients are considered to be adult learners ranging in ages from 16 to 45. Mrs. Young has had success as an educator and frequently receives positive feedback from her learners.

  6. According to Ms. Young, the first step in planning any educational
     training program is to: (p. 308)

        a. advertise and market the program

b. write objectives for the program
* c. do a needs assessment to determine if a need for the program exists.
d. gather the materials necessary to implement the program

7. Mrs. Young is planning an orientation program for new nursing staff; therefore, she would apply all of the following concepts <u>except</u>: (p. 317-318)

* a. utilize only one-way communication techniques such as lecture and assigned readings
b. allow the learners to plan and carry out their own learning experiences
c. utilize problem centered experiences rather than those that are theoretically oriented
d. allow the learners to apply and test their learning quickly
e. utilize a climate of openness and respect

<u>Situation 2</u>

Ms. Young is responsible for all inservice education for the obstetrical nursing staff. Staff include registered nurses and nursing assistants. Staff inservicing involves orientation, on-the-job training programs and staff enrichment. Since turnover of staff is high, Ms. Young keeps very busy with her job responsibilities.

8. Ms. Young has decided to utilize the preceptor model to orient new RN staff members. The role of a preceptor includes which of the following? (p. 318)

    a. orienter and teacher
    b. resource person and role model
    c. counselor
    d. evaluator
* e. all of the above

9. Ms. Young wants to evaluate on-the-job training programs in order to improve the quality of the program. Which of the following criteria would <u>not</u> be considered necessary to determine program effectiveness? (p. 323-324)

    a. trainee reaction questionnaire
    b. learning criteria to assess knowledge
    c. behavior change
    d. organizational impact
* e. client satisfaction

10. Learning requires at minimum: (p. 314)

    a. practice and transfer training
* b. practice and feedback
    c. modeling, practice, and reinforcement

d. attention, practice, and transfer
e. all of the above

11. Which of the following is not a learning transfer enhancer. (p. 311)

    a. identical elements
    b. adequate practice
    c. variety of stimuli
  * d. symbolic coding
    e. use of general principles
    f. reinforcement

12. An increase in production or a decrease in turnover in a department following training of the supervisor might serve as a _____ in evaluating the training. (pp. 323-324)

  * a. results criterion
    b. learning criterion
    c. behavioral criterion
    d. reaction criterion

13. For which of the following training situations would you recommend behavior modeling as a major instructional method? (pp. 312-314)

    a. a refresher course for typists
    b. an apprentice program for lathe operators
    c. an orientation program for new employees
  * d. a basic course in first-level supervision
    e. none of the above

14. The first step a trainer should take when training employees is: (p. 310)

  * a. gain attention
    b. give feedback
    c. use reinforcement
    d. present stimuli
    e. both c and d

15. The type of practice generally accepted as most efficient is: (pp. 310-311)

    a. massed
  * b. spaced
    c. mixed
    d. continuous
    e. none of the above

16. Problems of transfer of training arise in situations in which: (p. 311)

    a. the trainee has to change the rate of learning
    b. a new instructor is introduced into the training situation

124

* c. the trainee is given practice on a task that is not part of the actual job
  d. the trainee has to learn more than one set of skills to perform the job
  e. all of the above

ESSAY QUESTIONS:

17. How do people learn?

    Look for discussion of readiness to learn, motivation to learn, conditions for practice, transfer, memory span, social learning theory, relapse theory and adult education theory.
    (pp. 310-316)

18. Describe Social Learning Theory in detail.

    See Figure 14-3, and pp. 312-314

19. Explain the relapse process and what to do about it.

    See Figure 14-4, and p. 314-315

20. List as many training techniques as you can, then pick a training objective, state it, and tell me what technique you would use to meet the objective and why.

    This is an open question

21. Discuss the needs assessment process and how it is conducted.

    This topic is not discussed in the text. See p. 306.
    Needs analysis should include the following data collection techniques:

    a. organizational analysis to determine if there are constraints to the training and what resources are available
    b. task analysis to determine how to do the job
    c. person analysis to determine how the target population is currently doing the job
       Task and person analysis data are compared to determine performance deficiency. If the deficiency is one of skill rather than motivation and if training is a more logical intervention than selection, there is a training need.

22. Discuss the importance of the evaluation of training programs. Why is evaluation often ignored? Identify and discuss the four evaluative criteria. Relate each of these to the health care organization.

    a. It is important to determine if training caused any change or if trainees learned from a program. It is important to improve training programs and justify expenditures
    b. lack of money, time and/or ability to do it

c. trainee reaction, learning, behavior change, and   organizational result (pp. 321-324)

23. Discuss the principles of learning. Why should each of these principles be considered when developing training interventions? Discuss social learning theory.

    a. See pp. 310-316 for discussion of the following:
          learning principles
          readiness to learn
          motivation to learn
          practice
          whole vs. part learning
          spaced vs. massed practice
          overlearning
          transfer of training
          reinforcement/reward
          meaningfulness
          distinctiveness
          rehearsal
          grouping/checking/organization
    b. A training program must include the basic principles of learning to be successful.
    c. See Figure 14-3, p. 313

24. What is the preceptor model of staff orientation? Discuss the roles of the preceptor. How does the department of education influence the preceptor concept?

    a. Experienced staff nurses are selected on their clinical competence and teaching skills and then assist the new nurse to acquire necessary knowledge on the job
    b. See p. 318: orienter, teacher, resource person, counselor, role model and evaluator
    c. The department of education may provide initial orientation and training of preceptors (p. 317-321)

25. Discuss the need for patient education. What are the responsibilities of the nursing manager? What factors limit the effectiveness of patient education? Discuss how these limitations may be minimized.

    a. Due to shortened hospital stays, increase in long-term illness, to maintain health, to reduce malpractice suits, JCAHO standards
    b. to ensure staff is prepared, to document what is being done, assessment, to be aware of hospital-wide programs, and to help plan activities
    c. lack of priority
       lack of time
       lack of communication
       lack of skill
       lack of family involvement
       lack of continuity
         poor motivation

patient's physical condition
patient's psychosocial adaption and illness
(See pp. 324-329)

26. Discuss the importance of staff development. What is the role of the nursing manager in staff orientation? Describe on-the-job training. What are the key behaviors of on-the-job training? How can the nursing manager improve the effectiveness of on-the-job training?

    a. this is an open question
    b. see question 8 and p. 318
    c. see figure 14-6, p. 321
    d. see figure 14-6, p. 321
    e. see figure 14-7, p. 322

CHAPTER 15 - ENHANCING EMPLOYEE PERFORMANCE

TRUE/FALSE:

1. Motivation and ability are factors that influence job performance.

2. The first step in dealing with performance problems is to plan strategies for intervening with the specific employee problem.

3. Motivation factors that influence employee performance include selection and training.

4. The goal of day-to-day coaching is to deal with problems when they first occur and while they are still small and manageable.

5. From time to time, the nurse manager will be required to deal with rule violations which should be approached in an immediate forthright manner.

6. While the exact number of chemically dependent nurses is unknown, as many as one in ten to twenty graduates may experience the problem at some point in their career.

7. The impact of chemical dependency on the nurse's professional practice increases the risk of malpractice and of disciplinary action by the state licensing board.

8. It is easy for the nurse manager to identify staff who are chemically dependent.

9. When chemical dependency is identified, plans should be made for intervention. Intervention preparation should include collecting behavioral indicators of the problem as well as sources of help and treatment. When prepared, the appropriate personnel should meet with the nurse who is suspected to have a chemical dependency problem and confront the nurse with signs and symptons identified.

10. The least important intervention when dealing with a chemically dependent employee is to provide appropriate resources for counseling or support.

Answers:

        1. True,   Ch. 15, p. 334
        2. False,   p. 337
        3. False,   p. 337
        4. True,   p. 339
        5. True,   p. 341
        6. True,   pp. 342-343
        7. True,   pp. 342-343
        8. False,   p. 342

        9. True,   pp. 344-346
        10. False,   pp. 344-346

MULTIPLE CHOICES:

11. Which of the following would be <u>least</u> likely to act as a motivator for staff nurses? (p. 335)

      a. interest in producing high quality services
      b. a performance-based reward system
*   c. across-the-board yearly salary increases

12. Which of the following institutions is <u>most likely</u> to experience relatively <u>low levels</u> of employee absenteeism? (p. 335)

      a. those with no maximum number of sick days
*   b. those requiring notification of the supervisor in order to be paid for sick days
      c. those whose policy causes "loss" of sick days when an employee resigns
      d. those whose policy does not allow accrual of sick days

13. Which of the following are likely to lead to decreased productivity? (p. 336)

*   a. alcohol and substance abuse
      b. job enrichment
      c. sensitivity to employee needs
      d. task challenge

14. Which of the following is most important to successful performance?

      a. leadership
*   b. matching abilities and job requirements
      c. motivation
      d. organizational resources

15. Which of the following strategies promote congruence between ability and job requirements? (p. 337)

      a. recruitment efforts directed toward graduates of successful programs
      b. selection of employees based upon job requirements
      c. opportunity for continuing education
*   d. all of the above

16. Staff motivation is influenced by all <u>except</u>: (pp. 334-337)

      a. the compensation system
      b. benefits program
      c. style of supervision
      d. methods of selection
*   e. skill deficiencies

17. Job satisfaction is important because its components may influence productivity. These may include which of the following? (p. 337)

a. interpersonal relations
b. achievement
c. the work itself
d. recognition
* e. all of the above

18. In order for nurse managers to improve their appraisal accuracy skills, they must do all of the following except: (pp. 337-339)

   * a. rely upon their own absolute judgment rather than recognized guidelines
   b. record noteworthy behaviors throughout the evaluation period
   c. know what behaviors are contained in the employee's job description
   d. decide whether problems are skill or motivation related
   e. begin with accepted standards of performance

19. The primary purpose of discipline is to: (p. 341)

   a. punish employees for poor work performance
   * b. enhance employee performance and productivity
   c. allow supervisors to exercise proper authority in the work place
   d. set an example so that other employees will meet organizational "behavior sets".

20. Performance is a function of: (p. 337)

   a. ability and desire
   b. need, strength and ability
   c. ability and intrinsic motivation
   d. motivation x aptitude
   * e. ability x motivation

21. Which of the following statements regarding chemical dependency is incorrect? (pp. 342-344)

   a. 67% of all cases handled by state boards of nursing are related to alcohol or drug abuse
   b. Nurses whose licenses are sanctioned represent only a small portion of those who are addicted to alcohol and drugs.
   c. Nurses' professional fitness and lives are jeopardized when they become addicted
   * d. There has always been readily available help to assist chemically dependent nurses with recovery

22. Which of the following is not a true statement regarding the issue of chemical dependence? (p. 342)

   a. Professional functioning is impaired by chemical dependence
   b. Patients are put at risk when cared for by a chemically dependent nurse

130

  c. Staff morale may suffer when staff must carry a heavier workload due to absenteeism of the chemically dependent nurse
* d. Other staff members are generally not affected when working with a chemically dependent nurse

23. The <u>primary</u> symptom generally portrayed by the chemically dependent nurse is: (p. 342)

  a. irritability
* b. denial
  c. diaphoresis
  d. weight loss

<u>Situation 1</u>

A manager strongly suspects that there is a chemically dependent female nurse working on her unit. The nurse has had some absenteeism, has signed out narcotics as wasted on two occasions, and has become careless about her personal appearance.

24. The nurse manager's first action should be to: (p. 343)

  a. immediately approach the chemically dependent nurse and terminate her
  b. call all of the staff together and notify them of the situation
* c. investigate further to assess the situation, then take action
  d. fire her

25. Once the manager has identified that the nurse does in fact have a chemical abuse problem, the manager should first: (p. 344)

* a. inform her supervisor of the situation
  b. report the nurse to the State Board of Nursing
  c. check on health insurance provisions for chemical dependency treatments
  d. fire her

<u>Situation 2</u>

The chemically dependent nurse has agreed to enter treatment and is now recovering. She is ready for reentry into the work place. She has signed a contingency contract agreeing to abide by an agreement which states that she will attend a self-help recovery group, meet weekly with her supervisor regarding job performance, and submit to random urine screening for drugs and alcohol.

26. In preparing for re-entry the nurse manager should be involved in planning. Which of the following actions would most likely be considered to be in the best interest of the recovering nurse? (pp. 346-347)

  a. to place her on a different unit and allow her to administer drugs and narcotics

b. to retain her on the same unit and allow her to administer mood
       altering medications
 * c. to reassign her for a period of time to a unit or a task where no
       mood altering drugs are given

27. The staff on the unit where the recovering nurse has returned is unaware
    of the situation and the recovering nurse does not wish for them to know
    of her problem. Their jobs will not be affected in any way by the nurse's
    reentry. Who has the right to make the decision of whether or not the
    staff is to be told? (p. 347)

       a. the supervisor
       b. the head nurse
 * c. the recovering nurse in consultation with
       the treatment counselor
       d. administration

ESSAY QUESTIONS:

28. Identify factors that may increase motivation and employee
    productivity.

       compensation
       benefits program
       job design
       supervisory style
       recruiting/selection methods
       See pp. 334-337, Figure 15-1

29. How may employee ability serve as a deterrent to performance?

       See p. 336

30. Describe the key behaviors in diagnosing and remedying performance
    problems.

       See Figure 15-2, p. 338

31.   What steps should the nurse manager follow in dealing with a rule
       violation.

       See Figure 15-4, p. 341

32. In addition to individual signs and symptoms of chemical dependency, what
    signs on the unit should the nurse manager look for?

       See p. 342-344

33. What is the primary symptom of chemical dependency, and how does the nurse
    manager deal with it?

       a. denial by the nurse and other staff

b. investigate and take action (pp. 342-346)

34. Discuss the process of intervention with the chemically dependent nurse.
    a. examine institutional policies
    b. prepare for intervention
       collect all documentation
    c. obtain appropriate resources
          EAP or other counselor, AA
          support group
          health insurance
    d. examine own attitudes
    e. intervene
          small group, no interruptions
          focus on problem, not person
          take nurse directly to treatment if possible
          (p. 344-346)

35. Discuss reentry of the chemically dependent nurse.
    a. determine where to assign nurse
    b. develop and sign a contingency contract
    c. monitor returning nurse
    d. deal with staff concerns (p. 346-347)

CHAPTER 16 - PERFORMANCE APPRAISAL

TRUE/FALSE

1. Performance evaluation is often seen as a necessary evil which most nurse managers would rather avoid.

2. In recent years, evaluations have moved from behavior-based criteria to trait-based criteria in response to legal problems associated with behavior-based criteria.

3. Among problems resulting from evaluations is leniency error where the evaluator gives inflated ratings to some nurses.

4. The goal of day-to-day coaching is to deal with problems when they first occur and while they are still small and manageable.

5. From time to time, disciplinary action will be necessary; the action taken must be administered fairly and consistently.

Answers:

1. True, p. 350
2. False, pp. 351-352
3. False, pp. 358-359
4. True, p. 368
5. True, pp. 368-369

MULTIPLE CHOICE:

Situation 1
Kelly Bach, a B.S.N. graduate, has just completed an orientation for nurse manager on a surgical unit on which she has been working for the past five years. She is presently receiving coaching from her supervisor, Ms. Apple, regarding the writing of employee performance appraisals.

6. Ms. Apple has explained to Kelly that the performance appraisal process includes all of the following functions on her part except: (pp. 351-364)

     a. day-by-day interactions with her subordinates in the form of coaching, counseling, and disciplining
     b. written documentation of critical incidents and completion of the performance review form
*   c. formulation of a philosophy concerning performance appraisal which recognizes that the majority of employees will do minimum work
     d. the formal performance appraisal interview with follow-up sessions

7. Kelly is learning that the performance appraisal record is important because it may influence all of the following administrative decisions except: (p. 351)

     a. personnel salary increases
     b. personnel promotion

        c. personnel transfers
*   d. employee development
        e. personnel terminations

Situation 2

Nursing service and the personnel department are in the process of having managers and their staff submit data for a performance appraisal form for each classification of employee working on each hospital unit. Kelly's responsibility is to gather input from her staff regarding their preference of content and format for a performance appraisal form to submit to the personnel department for further development.

8. Kelly discusses the various methods of performance appraisal with her staff. Which of the following methods will both employees and supervisors have the most faith in and be motivated to use?

        a. essay evaluation
        b. traditional rating scales
        c. forced distribution evaluation
*   d. behavior-oriented rating scales
        e. management by objectives

9. Kelly is anxious to improve her appraisal accuracy skills. In order to do so she must do all of the following except: (pp. 360-361)

*   a. rely upon her own absolute judgment when completing the performance appraisal
        b. record noteworthy behaviors throughout the evaluation period
        c. know what behaviors are contained in the employee's job description
        d. observe the employee's performance over the entire period of evaluation
        e. know how to use the appraisal form and understand what is meant by each performance dimension

10. A manager sees that a subordinate always writes excellent reports. At appraisal time, he rates her high on this dimension and high on all the other dimensions even though she is constantly late, a poor speaker, and very argumentative. This is an example of: (p. 359)

        a. stereotyping
*   b. halo error
        c. projection
        d. accuracy

11. Mary Nelson has six subordinates and she has a large scope and depth of responsibilities. She really had little time for performance appraisal so she rated all six as average. This error is known as: (p. 358)

        a. recency bias
        b. halo error
        c. leniency

```
    * d. central tendency
      e. association
```

12. Comparing an individual's job performance against standards or objectives developed for the individual's position is known as: (pp. 355-357)

```
      a. a job description
      b. a job evaluation
      c. a job specification
    * d. performance evaluation
      e. orientation
```

13. The primary purpose of discipline is to: (pp. 368-369)

```
      a. punish employees for poor work performance
    * b. encourage employees to behave sensibly at work
      c. allow supervisors to exercise proper authority in the work place
      d. set an example, so that other employees will meet organizational
         "behavior sets".
```

14. Performance is a function of: (pp. 360-361)

```
      a. ability and desire
      b. need, strength and ability
      c. ability and intrinsic motivation
      d. motivation x aptitude
    * e. ability x motivation
```

15. Whatever the level of the standards employed by a given superior, there is a possibility that he will rate all subordinates within a narrow range at the middle of the scale. This is called: (p. 358)

```
      a. halo error
      b. constant error
      c. recency error
    * d. central tendency error
      e. personal bias
```

16. Each of the following is an organizational goal for performance appraisal except: (pp. 351-351)

```
      a. providing the employee with feedback.
      b. influencing the employee's performance
    * c. enhancing the organizational climate
      d. gathering data for the organization
      e. providing the individual with counseling.
```

17. The appraisal interview is used in connection with:
```
      a. hiring employees
    * b. improving individual performance
      c. job placement
      d. labor-turnover analysis
```

<u>ESSAY QUESTIONS</u>:

18. Compare and contrast absolute and comparative judgement rating scales.

    See Figure 16-1 and 16-2, pp. 363-366

19. Describe and discuss the key behaviors for performance reviews given in the text.

    See Figure 16-4 and discussion, pp. 366-368

20. How may the results of performance appraisal be used? What are the legal issues associated with the uses of performance appraisal? Discuss the guidelines which, if followed, increase the legal defensibility of the performance appraisal.

    a. for administrative decisions (salary increases, promotions, transfers), to tie rewards to performance, for employee feedback and development, to conform to EEO Law, and to use as criteria in selection system validation studies (p. 360)
    b. See list, p. 351
    c. See list, p. 351

21. Identify and discuss the specific methods of evaluation. What are the strengths and weaknesses of each? Which is/are most appropriate for nursing?

    a/b. traditional rating scales (p. 355)
        essay evaluation (p. 355)
        forced distribution (p. 355-356)
        BOS (p. 357)
        MBO (p. 357)
    c. open question, probably BOS

22. Identify those individuals who are potential evaluators. Who appears to be the most appropriate evaluator of the nurse's performance? Why?

    a. immediate supervisor, co-workers, the employee herself, patients/family, other supervisors
    b. criteria:
    Who has the information?
    Who has the motivation to rate accurately?
    Who has the ability?
    Best answer: head nurse (pp. 357-358)

23. There are several types of performance rating error. Identify and discuss each. How may these sources of error be lessened?

    a. leniency error (p. 358)
        recency error (p. 359)
        halo error (p. 359)
        ambiguous evaluation standards (p. 359)

written comments problem (p. 360)
   b. all can be lessened by increasing rater ability and motivation (p. 360-361)

24. Discuss the importance of documenting employee performance. Describe one method of documentation.

   a. It is important to document employee performance to enhance rater memory, make writing the appraisal easier, and for EEO law. (p. 361)
   b. noteworthy or critical incidents (p. 361-364)

25. Discuss the performance appraisal interview. How does the evaluator/ nursing manager prepare for the interview? What are the key behaviors of the evaluator/nursing manager for the performance appraisal interview?

   a. look for why it is done (see question 3)
   b. review appraisal form and critical incidents
         understand employee
         anticipate potential disagreement
         advance notice
         prepare specific examples of behavior
         prepare private setting with ample time (pp. 364-366)
   c. See Figure 16-4, p. 366

26. Identify and discuss the key behaviors of day-to-day coaching. Why is day-to-day coaching important? When should the nursing manager use coaching rather than discipline?

   a. See Figure 15-3, p. 339 and discussion p. 368-370.
   b. to correct performance deficiencies, employee development
   c. Always use coaching at least once before discipline. (p. 370)

27. Identify and discuss the key behaviors of disciplining employees. Identify some guidelines for effective disciplining.

   See Figure 16-5, pp. 368 & 370

CHAPTER 17 - UNDERSTANDING AND MANAGING NURSE ABSENTEEISM AND TURNOVER

TRUE/FALSE

1. Employee absenteeism and turnover pose serious problems for the health care industry.

2. According to the Rhoades and Steers model, employee absenteeism is a function of the individual's ability to attend and motivation to attend.

3. The way in which the nurse manager can exercise the most influence on absenteeism is by affecting the staff's ability to attend.

4. Dysfunctional turnover such as the loss of a highly skilled nurse who will be hard to replace can be expensive as well as negatively affect the unit's morale.

5. The nurse manager can decrease voluntary turnover by influencing the staff nurse's perception of ease of movement (to a limited degree) and the desirability of movement (to a great degree).

Answers:

    1. True, Ch. 17, p. 373
    2. True,   p. 373
    3. False,   p. 375
    4. True,   p. 383-387
    5. True,   p. 385

MULTIPLE CHOICE:

6. Which of the following influences an employee's ability to attend? (pp.374-375)

        a. work group norms
        b. employee values and job expectations
        c. supervisors' leadership styles
    *   d. family responsibilities
        e. opportunity for upward mobility

7. When considering applicants, which of the following approaches should be employed by the nurse manager who is attempting to reduce absenteeism on her nursing unit? (p. 377-378)

        a. inquire about the applicant's marital status
        b. ask the applicant about arrangements for child care
    *   c. review the applicant's previous absenteeism record
        d. review personal characteristics that might increase susceptibility to illness

8. Absenteesm may be reduced or controlled by all of the following except: (p. 377-379)

     a. evaluation of attendance during the employees' performance appraisal
     b. increasing staff awareness of the costs of absenteeism
 * c. adoption of an institutional policy whereby unused sick days will be lost
     d. allocation of merit pay for good attendance
     e. peer pressure on absence-prone staff

9. Which of the following institutional policies would be least likely to reduce absenteeism and promote satisfaction over a long period of time? (p. 377-379)

 * a. sanctions to discourage absenteeism
     b. placing no limit on the number of sick days that can accumulate
     c. credit for unused sick days in determining retirement   date
     d. conversion of a specified number of unused sick days to vacation days

10. When attempting to control involuntary turnover, which of the following factors should the nurse manager explore further when interviewing an applicant for a nursing position? (p. 385-387)

     a. the applicant's realistic understanding of the   position's requirements
 * b. the applicant's experience in several previous   positions
     c. interest in upward and lateral mobility
     d. the applicant's child care responsibilities

11. Voluntary turnover may be decreased by which of the following?

     a. an employee's perceived ease of leaving
     b. an employee's desirability of leaving
     c. dissatisfaction with the job situation
 * d. opportunity for position transfer within the institution

Situation 1

A general hospital has experienced an increase in voluntary turnover in nursing positions. Variability in patient census often requires staff nurses to work overtime or to change scheduled days off in order to provide adequate staffing.

12. Which of the following conditions would contribute to dysfunctional turnover at this general hospital? (p. 382-383)

     a. the lack of vested pension by a departing nurse
     b. mediocre performance by a departing nurse manager
 * c. superior performance by a departing staff nurse

d. financial savings resulting from the salary difference between departing and replacement employee

13. If this hospital is forced to consider discontinuing positions because of many low census days, which of the following pressure-to-attend work factors would most likely influence a staff nurse's attendance? (p. 377-379)

    a. personal work ethic
* b. fear of losing one's position
    c. work group norms
    d. organizational commitment

Situation 2

After several months the patient census and patient acuity levels at the general hospital have increased and the hospital is now experiencing a nursing shortage. Registered nurses are expected to work when and where they are needed. Employee turnover continues to increase.

14. Which of the following is <u>least</u> likely to account for the increased turnover of registered nurses in this hospital?
(pp. 381-385)

    a. nurses are working shorthanded
    b. non-work activities are interrupted by overtime and working scheduled days off
* c. satisfaction with the quality of patient care has increased
    d. nurses are physically and mentally exhausted
    e. nursing units are being closed when adequate care cannot be provided

15. The nurse manager needing to control absenteeism of her staff at this general hospital would most appropriately:
(pp. 377-378)

    a. provide a written warning to any staff nurse who is absent regardless of the cause
* b. analyze the satisfaction of her staff nurses with their job situation
    c. explore ways to enrich the position of the staff nurse
    d. discourage the legitimate use of sick days

ESSAY QUESTIONS:

16. Discuss Rhoades and Steers model of attendance/absenteeism behavior. What are the two main variables of this model?

    a. See Figure 17-1 and discussion (pp. 374-376)
    b. ability to attend and motivation to attend (p. 374)

17. Discuss the differences between voluntary and involuntary absenteeism. Discuss attempts to measure each.

    a. voluntary is personal business and involuntary is sickness or transportation problems. The distinction is fine in theory but difficult in practice. (p. 373)
    b. absence frequency vs. total days absent, see p. 374

18. What are some examples of costs of absenteeism within nursing?

    cost of replacement
    cost of short staffing on other staff (p. 373)

19. Discuss potential action the nursing manager may take to decrease absenteeism.

    understand it
    establish climate which discourages abuse of sick days
    study absence patterns
    coaching/performance appraisal
    motivate staff to attend (pp. 377-378)

20. Discuss potential action the hospital may take to decrease absenteeism.

    childcare centers
    sick leave policy
    shuttle buses/car pools
    stress reduction programs
    include attendance in performance appraisal
    (pp. 377-380)

21. Using Rhoades and Steers model, discuss how absenteeism may be controlled. Which of the two major variables that affect absenteeism does the organization have more control over?

    a. see questions 4 and 5 and pp. 344-376
    b. motivation to attend

22. Identify and discuss the different types of turnover. From the organization's point of view, what are the consequences of each type of turnover?

    a. voluntary and involuntary - see p. 381
       functional or dysfunctional - see p. 382
    b. involuntary - get rid of poor employee
       voluntary - may be good employee or bad employee
       functional - lose poor employee
       dysfunctional - lose good employee (see pp. 382-383)

23. What direct and indirect turnover control measures are available to the nursing manager?

analyze who leaves and who stays - hire the "stayers"
improve <u>all</u> working conditions
improve pay and benefits
allow internal transfer
work on job satisfaction
avoid "quick fixes"
reward good performance
be concerned with work scheduling (p. 385-387)

24. Discuss categories of reasons for leaving

See Figure 17-3

CHAPTER 18 - NURSING ASSOCIATIONS AND COLLECTIVE BARGAINING

TRUE/FALSE

1. Unionization in the health care field is growing despite an overall decline in union membership in the United States.

2. In order to change contract terms in a health care institution, notification in writing within 60 days and not less than 30 days prior to the expiration date of the agreement, is required by law. This measure allows time for contingency planning in the event a strike is called.

3. Collective bargaining decreases the strength of the individual worker.

4. Grievances usually result from: 1) misunderstandings, 2) intentional contract violations, or 3) symptomatic problems outside the confines of the labor agreement.

5. Symptomatic grievances have three basic causes: 1) personal problems, 2) union politics, or 3) unfavorable contract language.

6. In Canada, most nurses belong to a union which negotiates in their behalf during contract disputes.

7. The Rand Formula ensures a continuous and predictable income for the union by requiring mandatory payment of union dues.

8. Independent nursing unions affiliated with trade unions are a distinctive feature of the nursing profession in Canada.

Answers:

    1. True, p. 392
    2. False, p. 394
    3. False, p. 395
    4. True, p. 397
    5. True, p. 398
    6. True, p. 400
    7. True, p. 402
    8. False, p. 404

MULTIPLE CHOICE:

Situation 1

As a relatively new nurse manager, Susan realizes the need to increase her knowledge base concerning nursing associations and collective bargaining when she is advised to drop her membership in the American Nurses Association because she is now a part of administration.

 9. Why may Susan's membership in the American Nurses Association present a problem if she is part of the administrative staff?
    (p. 397)

* a. Her membership may be viewed as a conflict of interest if the
        association serves as the bargaining agent for her subordinates.
     b. Nurses believe the professional organization should not serve as a
        labor organization and that this dualism represents a conflict of
        professional purposes and standards
     c. Nurses believe that there is no conflict and that the promotion
        of nurses' economic security and general welfare is a major
        responsibility of the organization.

10. Collective bargaining looks increasingly attractive to nurses for all of
    the following reasons except: (p. 396)

     a. frustration about the inability to practice nursing as they
        believe it should be practiced
     b. to gain improved personnel policies and benefits
     c. to improve and influence working conditions
   * d. to attain professional autonomy and control of the working
        environment

Situation 2

As a nurse manager in a private, not-for-profit hospital which is unionized,
Susan must learn the nurse manager's role in administering the union contract
with regard to her unit staff.

11. The nurse manager's role includes all of the following except:
    (pp. 397-398)

     a. actively helping to administer the grievance procedure
     b. adhering to negotiated working hours for staff
   * c. formulating and presenting suggested staff wage increases to
        nursing service administration
     d. actively participating in issues related to discipline

12. Susan has a union manual containing the usual classified grievances.
    All of the following are included except: (p. 397)

     a. misunderstanding
     b. intentional contract violation
     c. symptomatic problems
   * d. wage increase negotiations

13. Which major federal law protects individual employees in their
    exercise of union activities? (p. 392)

   * a. Wagner Act
     b. Landrum Griffin Act
     c. Taft-Hartley Act
     d. Norris-LaGuardia Act
     e. Civil Rights Act

14. The union that wins a representative election has which of the
    following duties and rights? (pp. 392-397)

a. The duty to represent only union members in the bargaining unit
b. The right to forbid management from unilaterally changing employment conditions for employees outside the bargaining unit.
c. The right to jointly negotiate expanded bargaining units with the employer after the election.
* d. None of the above.

15. Which of the following are bargainable, according to the National Labor Relations Act? (pp. 392-394)

a. wages
b. hours
c. working conditions
* d. all of the above

16. The cornerstone of effective labor-management relations is: (p. 393)

* a. bargaining in good faith
b. an honest union election
c. ability to resolve complaints before grievances are filed
d. ability to agree on every proposal

17. Employer unfair labor practices include all but which of the following: (p. 393)

a. coercing employees
b. telling employees the hospital will close
c. discriminating against employees for union activities
d. refusing to bargain in good faith
* e. all are unfair labor practices

18. Which of the following issues appears not to be significantly related to a willingness to favor union representation? (p. 395)

a. job security
* b. challenging work
c. supervisory practices
d. wages

19. Which of the following examples of bargaining issues must management agree to discuss upon union request? (p. 393)

a. product prices
b. production schedules
* c. 32-hour work weeks
d. all of the above
e. none of the above

20. Major differences between the U.S. and Canadian approaches to labor legislation according to Carter are all of the following except: (pp. 402-403)

    a. certification process
    b. strike restrictions
    c. compulsory grievance arbitration
    d. recognition of the right to union security
 * e. accreditation process

21. In Canadian provinces where strikes by hospitals are prohibited, negotiations for compulsory binding arbitration are referred to which of the following: (pp. 402-404)

 * a. independent boards
    b. the bargaining agent
    c. the employer

Situation 3

Staff nurses, employed at a hospital, are represented by an independent union organization. They are now in the process of negotiation concerning their grievances.

22. Since the staff nurses belong to an independent union organization, which of the following statements is correct? (p. 405)

    a. they may not also belong to the professional nursing association
 * b. they may also belong to the professional nursing association
    c. they may belong to only one association at a time

23. The staff nurses are seriously considering a strike as negotiations are reaching an impasse. Which of the following is not a true statement regarding strikes? (pp. 401-402)

    a. strikes are generally regarded as the ultimate economic sanction that can be exercised by a union
 * b. strikes are allowed in order to gain recognition as a bargaining agent

    c. a strike vote must be taken before a union is entitled to a strike

    d. a formal notice of a strike must be given to the employer

ESSAY QUESTIONS:

24. Discuss health care labor relations. Which hospitals are subject to jurisdiction under U.S. labor law?

    a. open question; See question #1

b. private, non-profit hospitals, nursing homes, clinics, and HMO's;
    all proprietary health care facilities (p. 392)

25. How do the 1974 health care amendments influence union activity? Discuss
    how unionization has influenced health care.

    a. Union activity is legal and regulated. Union membership has
        increased (pp. 392-394)
    b. This is an open question; (pp. 394-395)

26. Discuss the impact of unionization on wages and hospital costs.
    (see pp. 394-395)

27. What are the major provisions of the Wagner Act?

    Section 7 - employee rights
    unfair labor practices
    union organization election procedure (pp. 392-393)

28. Discuss the relationship between nursing professional associations and
    unions. What are the pros and cons associated with membership in each of
    these organizations?

    See discussion of SNA's, p. 395-397
    conflict between unionization and professionalism
    conflict between union status and supervisory position
    See pp. 395-397

29. Discuss the grievance process. Review the suggestions for handling
    grievances. What are the key behaviors to be followed in the grievance
    hearing?

    steps of the process, p. 398
    See list on pp. 398-400.
    See list on p. 400.

30. What are the major differences between the Canadian and U.S. approaches to
    labor legislation? How may the nurse manager in a Canadian hospital
    behave with a unionized staff as compared to his/her American counterpart?
        See pp. 400-404

31. What is the history of collective bargaining by Canadian nurses?
    Discuss the relationship between professional nursing associations and
    unions. (pp. 403-404)

32. What are the strike restrictions in Canadian collective bargaining?

    a. cannot be used to gain recognition
    b. except in Saskatchewan, not allowed while an agreement is in
        effect

c. must use certain mediation/conciliation process before striking while negotiating a contract and a formal notice of a strike must be given to employer
d. not allowed in Prince Edward Isle, Newfoundland, Ontario, and Alberta except by public health nurses (pp. 401-402)

CHAPTER 19 - BUDGETING AND RESOURCE ALLOCATION

TRUE/FALSE

1. Increasingly, a nurse manager must become proficient in budgetary control as nursing expenditures can be up to half of a hospital's total budget.

2. The most effective budgets are prepared by management without input from staff personnel. These budgets tend to cause less friction than those where employees are active in the budgetary process.

3. When considering a capital purchase, the nurse manager should consider how much money it will cost to maintain the routine operations during the fiscal year.

4. Zero-base budgeting requires justification of all expenditures each budgetary period rather than beginning with the budget from the previous period.

5. The personnel budget can account for up to 90% of the total nursing budget; it includes items such as salaries, sick leave, vacation pay and overtime pay.

Answers:

        1. True, p. 410
        2. False, p. 414
        3. False, p. 416
        4. True, p. 414
        5. True, p. 419

MULTIPLE CHOICE:

6. A unit personnel budget can be developed by all of the following except:
    (p. 420)

        a. predicting patient days by level of activity
        b. determining hours of nursing care required for the patient mix
      * c. distributing hours required over two shifts
        d. developing a staffing pattern considering personnel mix available
        e. converting hours of care to actual costs

7. The personnel budget is influenced by all of the following except:
    (pp. 419-425)

        a. patient census
        b. acuity levels
        c. technology changes
        d. changes in medical practice
      * e. zero-base budgeting

8. A total unit budget includes all of the following budgets except:
    (p. 415-419)

* a. flexible budget
  b. personnel budget
  c. supply and expense budget
  d. capital expenditure budget

9. All of the following statements concerning the <u>capital</u> <u>expenditure</u> <u>budget</u> are true <u>except</u>:

    a. it funds the purchase of major equipment
    b. it provides money for architectural renovations
    c. nurse managers keep a chronological listing of all capital items purchased
  * d. it provides money to purchase service contracts, medical and surgical supplies

10. The personnel budget can logically be expected to cover which of the following items? (p. 419)

    a. salaries of nursing staff
    b. vacation time staff
    c. sick leave staff
    d. day care for the pre-school children of nursing staff
    e. orientation of nursing staff
  * f. all of the above can be covered

11. When establishing a budgetary plan for a given staffing pattern on a nursing unit, the nurse manager must take into consideration all of the following variables <u>except</u>: (pp. 419-422)

  * a. vacation days
    b. personnel mix
    c. hours of work per shift
    d. distribution of work load
    e. delivery system used

<u>Situation 1</u>

Recently promoted nurse manager, Jane Bach, BSN-RN, is meeting with the hospital controller in order to learn her budgetary functional role.

12. Jane has learned that there are four types of budgets she needs to know in order to manage her unit effectively. They include all of the following <u>except</u>: (entire chapter)

  * a. the management budget
    b. the operating budget
    c. the capital expenditure budget
    d. the supply and expense budget
    e. units of service

<u>Situation 2</u>

Jane learns that nearly all hospital budgets are derived in some way and to some extent from the forecast of patient occupancy rates, acuity levels, or some other activity standard.

14. What is the unit of service upon which the budgetary concept for expenses is based? (p. 415)

      a. square footage per unit
   * b. patient days
      c. acuity of client
      d. third party payee

15. Jane is absolutely amazed when she learns the percentage of the total nursing service budget which will be allocated to the salaries of nursing service personnel. This allocation is: (p. 419)

      a. 50-60%
      b. 70-75%
   * c. 85-90%
      d. 80%
      e. the personnel budget

ESSAY QUESTIONS:

16. Identify the four types of budgets. What are the advantages and disadvantages of each? Identify those budget components with which the nursing manager is directly involved.

    a. capital expense budget
       supply and expense budget
       personnel budget
       operating budget (pp. 415-419)
    b. see p. 415-420; to increase efficiency, to monitor, to project costs, to communicate
    c. mostly the personnel budget, supply and expense budget (pp. 419-425)

17. What is the capital expenditure budget? What are two common criteria associated with the capital expenditure budget?

    a. to fund purchases of major equipment or architectural renovations over a certain cost or having an expected life
    b. $500 or above and one year life (p. 416)

18. Discuss the supply and expense budget. What steps should be followed in the development of a supply and expense budget? How is this budget monitored?

    a. funds noncapital equipment and supplies (p. 418)
    b. keep and monitor expense statements
       adjust for inflation
       adjust for expected acuity, census, new services
       communicate (pp. 418-419)

19. Discuss the process of personnel budget development. What factors are involved in developing a staffing pattern?

    a. predict patient days by level of acuity determine fixed vs. variable staffing calculate in all changes and regulatory requirements develop and review plans/goals for next year develop staffing pattern, FTE and positions covered assign FTE's, differentials, benefits and predicted overtime develop budget (pp. 419-425)
    b. personnel mix, hours of work, distribution of work load, and delivery system (p. 420)

20. What factors influence personnel budget planning? How may the nursing manager identify the extent to which each of these factors may be affecting the budget?

    a. See list p. 419.
    b. See p. 419-420.

21. Explain the effect of differentials and overtime on personnel budgeting.

    Differentials increase the personnel costs for evening and night shift, overtime must be established to cover situations that cannot be anticipated. (pp. 423-424)

22. Explain what a capital item request form is used for and what it looks like.

    See Figure 19-3, p. 417

23. Discuss variance reports.

    See Figure 19-2, p. 413

24. Discuss budgeting in terms of planning and controlling.

    Planning-   reviewing goals/objectives, establishing fiscal projections, communicating budget information, coordinating and monitoring budget compliance

    Control -   comparing actual expenses to budget, making modifications and corrections, monitoring budget compliance

25. Explain zero-base budgeting

    It requires managers to start from zero budget level each year and to justify all costs anew (p. 414)

26. Calculate the units of service for one year for a 30 bed nursing unit when the unit has a 75% occupancy rate.
    (See pp. 419-420)

27. Determine the daily hours of nursing care required if there are 15 "level II" patients requiring six hours of care per patient day. How are "total" hours of care for a 24-hour period determined? (See p. 420)

28. Calculate the number of variable FTE's required per day when the required nursing hours are 180 hours per 24 hours and each nurse works a eight hour shift. (see pp. 420-421)

CHAPTER 20 - MANAGING AND INITIATING CHANGE

TRUE/FALSE:

1. Change in health care is inevitable; nurses should strive to be leaders in that change rather than merely players controlled by others.

2. All systems produce stress and conflict because of the opposing forces of the system's maintenance and adaptive mechanisms. Maintenance mechanisms work to keep the system changing over time while adaptive mechanisms prevent change from occurring too quickly.

3. Whenever organizations change, an integrative approach should be used. This is true because regardless where the change begins, whether in technology, structure or people, the other two components will be affected.

4. Whenever change occurs you can anticipate generalized resistance. Change can be both positive and negative. On the positive side, resistance forces the change agents to be clear about why the change is needed. On the negative side, resistance can eventually wear down those working to bring about change.

5. Creative thinking and breaking out of traditional molds are not essential for nurses who want to be innovators in their field of expertise.

Answers:

    1. True, p. 428
    2. False, p. 428
    3. True, p. 430
    4. True, p. 443
    5. False, p. 446

MULTIPLE CHOICE:

Situation 1

Mrs. Hermann, a hospital inservice educator, is planning to present a series of five programs on "How to Stop Smoking" to a group of volunteer clients who wish to break the habit. The various sessions will include teaching methods such as lecture, audiovisual aids, and group discussions.

6. Since Mrs. Hermann will apply Lewin's process of change, the first intervention she will attempt is to: (p. 431)

    * a. unfreeze the existing equilibrium
      b. move the target system to a new level of equilibrium
      c. refreeze the system
      d. none of the above

7. Should Mrs. Hermann apply Lippitt's phases of change, her first step would be to: (p. 433)

        a. assess the client's motivation and capacity for change
        b. assess the change agent's motivation and resources
  * c. diagnose the problem
        d. none of the above

Situation 2

An OB clinical specialist routinely presents parenting classes one night per week to a group of eager prospective parents. They have signed up for the classes voluntarily and have paid a small fee.

8. Which change strategy would the clinician most likely choose for this particular group? (p. 441)

        a. power-coercive
  * b. empirical-rational
        c. normative-reeducative
        d. any will do

9. If the same clinical specialist was to present a class on "contraception" to a group which was basically opposed to any form of birth control, she may choose to use which strategy? (p. 441)

        a. power-coercive
  * b. normative-reeducative
        c. empirical-rational
        d. none of the above

10. Which of the following is not one of the major issues in organizational change? (p. 439)

        a. which approach to take
        b. the obvious problem may not be the real one
  * c   packaged courses are always worse than individualized programs
        d. top down or bottom up change
        e. radical vs. gradual change

11. What would you not do in introducing change to employees? (p. 433-440)

        a. tell them why the change is necessary
        b. make a radical change
        c. let the employees participate in designing the change schedule
        d. tell one subordinate to inform his peers about the change
  * e. both b and d

12. People avoid change because of: (p. 443)

        a. their ingrained personalities
        b. their need to maintain cognitive consistency
        c. selective exposure to people and ideas
  * d. all of the above

13. Which of the following is <u>not</u> an advantage in using the systems frame of reference to understand and manage change? (p. 429-430)

    a. it mandates integrative thinking
    b. it directs attention to the hierarchical arrangements of the institutions subsystems.
*   c. it forces the change agent to search for simple cause and effect relationships

14. Lewin's force field model of change includes: (pp. 431-432)

    a. restraining and driving forces
    b. unfreezing, moving and refreezing
    c. diagnosing, assessing, selecting objects, and choosing a charge agent role
    d. diffusion of innovations
    e. all of the above
*   f. a and b only

15. Having an employee who is resisting a change serve on a committee to develop a plan for change implementation is an example of: (p. 443-445)

    a. manipulation
    b. negotiation
*   c. cooptation
    d. coercion
    e. facilitation and support

16. Lewin's change process consists of which phases?

    a. planning, implementing, evaluating
    b. diagnosis, prognosis, treatment
*   c. unfreezing, moving, refreezing
    d. diagnosis, treatment prognosis
    e. thesis, antithesis, synthesis

<u>ESSAY QUESTIONS</u>:

17. What are the steps you should take in making an organizational change?

    a. identify the problem or opportunity
    b. collect data
    c. analyze data
    d. plan the change strategies
    e. implement the change
    f. evaluate the effectiveness
    g. stabilize the change (pp. 434-440)

18. Name three methods of organizational change aimed at individuals.

    information giving
    training

counseling/psychotherapy
selection/placement/termination (pp. 430, 439)

19. Why should you be the one to explain an organizational change to your subordinates?

  a. to maintain control, information, and credibility
  b. to create a supportive climate, act as energizer, obtain and provide feedback and overcome resistance (p. 430 and 439)

20. What should you do when you must assign a "badnews job" to a subordinate? Be succinct and list the steps. (p. 444)

21. Discuss the impact of DRGs on nursing and the changes in health care you see in the future.

    This is an evolving answer and not specifically answered in this chapter.

22. Discuss the notion of nurse manager as change agent.

    See change agent strategies, p. 440.
    See change agent skills, p. 442.
    See handling resistance, p. 443.
    See politics of change, p. 445.
Also:
    internal vs. external consultant
    nurses control quality of care, quality of care makes for a
        competitive edge
    nurses help control the cost of health care
    proactive rather than reactive

23. Why should you use a systems frame of reference to understand and manage change?

    most nurses work in complex organizations so a systems perspective is critical

    It mandates integrative thinking.
    Inhibits accepting simple casual relationships.
    Directs attention to hierarchical nature of organizations.
    It mandates a macro perspective (p. 429).

24. Describe at least three change theories.

    See pp. 431-434, and Figure 20-1

        Lewin's Force-Field Model
        Lippit's phases of change
        Havelock Model
        Roger's Diffusion of Innovations
        Text's Eclectic Approach

25. Describe the change agent strategies.

      power-coercive
      empirical-rational
      normative-reducative (pp. 440-442)

26. List the ten change agent skills as described in the text. (p. 114)

CHAPTER 21 - QUALITY ASSURANCE AND RISK MANAGEMENT

TRUE/FALSE:

1. Hospitals sustain liability in two forms of negligence. Custodial negligence occurs when patient injury results from the quality of care given. Professional negligence occurs when environmental conditions result in injury.

2. Quality assurance is a process for evaluating the quality of care given to patients. It includes setting standards, determining criteria, and evaluating performance as well as planning for change and follow-up.

3. As litigation has increased, risk management has grown in importance. Risk management is a program designed to reduce losses through prevention.

4. Incident reports are an essential part of risk management. Any unplanned or unexpected occurrences which may affect the patient or family should be reported.

5. Through prompt attention and care, the nurse manager can often avoid potential liability claims.

Answers:

        1. False, p. 450
        2. True, p. 451
        3. True, p. 454
        4. True, p. 457-460
        5. True, p. 461

MULTIPLE CHOICE:

Situation 1

Part of Mary Johnson's nurse management orientation program will be spent with Sheila East in the quality assurance department.

6. Sheila is explaining to Mary what her responsibilities for implementing the quality assurance process on her unit will be. All of the following are included except: (pp. 452-453)

        a. setting standards
        b. determining criteria
        c. evaluating performance
     * d. reporting nursing staff tardiness
        e. planning for change and evaluation

7. Mary has previously participated in monitoring nursing care by all of the following methods except: (p. 453-454)

        * a. serving as a member of the procedure committee
          b. nursing audit
          c. peer review
          d. utilization review
          e. patient satisfaction interviews

8. The term "quality assurance" can best be described as: (p. 452)

          a. optimum levels of care
          b. an examination or review of records
          c. a review of practices by an equal
        * d. an effort to evaluate and ensure quality health care.

9. The term "peer review" describes: (p. 454)

          a. optimum levels of care
          b. an examination or review of records
        * c. a review of practices by an equal
          d. an effort to evaluate and ensure quality health care

10. The BEST description of an "audit" would be: (p. 453-454)

          a. optimum levels of care
        * b. an examination or review of records
          c. a review of practices by an equal
          d. an effort to evaluate and ensure quality health care

Situation 2

Mrs. Hall has just delivered her first baby and is planning to breast feed.
The nurse formulates a nursing diagnosis of knowledge deficit related to
breast feeding. The outcome criterion is that the client will breast feed her
infant for 5 minutes from each breast within 48 hours of delivery.

11. After two days, Mrs. Hall is tearful and states, "I'll never be able to
    breast feed as long as my nipples are sore." This state is an example
    of: (p. 452)

        * a subjective data
          b. objective data
          c. outcome criterion
          d. a standard

12. The nurse makes the following entry on the nursing care plan: "Goal not
    met, client refuses to breastfeed due to dry, cracked nipples." Since
    the goal has not been met the nurse should: (pp. 452-454)

          a. reassign Mrs. Hall to another caregiver
        * b. reexamine nursing strategies
          c. notify the physician
          d. suggest Mrs. Hall bottle feed

13. During Mrs. Hall's hospitalization, the quality assurance nurse reviews the interventions that the nurses have documented on the client's chart. This is an example of a: (p. 454)

    a. terminal audit
*   b. concurrent audit
    c. retrospective audit
    d. valid audit

14. If the quality assurance nurse were to directly observe the nurses giving care to Mrs. Hall, this would be an audit of: (p. 454-456)

*   a. process
    b. outcome
    c. agency structure

ESSAY QUESTIONS:

15. Discuss the key behaviors of handling a complaint.

    See Figure 21-3, p. 462

16. How does the attitude of the nursing manager influence the risk management system?

    It is the nurse manager who sets the tone on the unit that contributes to a safe and low-risk environment. If the manager is supportive of staff who report patient incidences, they will be more likely to keep the manager informed about potential risk situations. (p. 449)

17. What is risk management? What are the components of a risk management program? How is a risk management program developed?

    a. a planned program of loss prevention and liability control
    b. identifying potential risks
       reviewing present institutional monitoring systems
       analyzing incidents
       reviewing procedures
       monitoring laws and codes
       eliminating/reducing risks
       reviewing work of other committees
       identifying patient needs
       evaluating the results
       providing reports
    c. see b. above (pp. 454-455)

18. Who are the members of a risk management committee? What are the responsibilities of the risk manager?

    a. See list, p. 455
    b. See list, p. 456

19. Discuss the risk management organization model.

       See Figure 21-1, p. 457

20. Discuss the importance of monitoring and analyzing incident reports. What are the benefits of a risk management program?

    a.   They serve to document institutional, nurse, and physician accountability. If at fault, the institution is more likely to get sued and lose.

    b.   Incident reports are used to analyze the severity, frequency and causes of incidents. Such analysis serves as a basis for intervention and prevention. (p. 457-460)

21. Discuss the process of reporting incidents.

       See list on p. 505 and Figure 21-2, p. 457-460

22. What are the areas of high risk in the health care organization? Which of these areas involves the department of nursing?

    a.   see list, p. 457
         examples can be found, p. 458-460
    b.   all five areas (p. 457)

23. What is the role of nursing in risk management? Discuss the process for reporting incidents and why nurses are reluctant to report incidents. What are some examples of risk incidents?

    a.   Nurses are involved in patient care 24 hours a day, involved in all risk categories. Nurses are critical to any risk management program success. (p. 454)

    b.   See list, p. 458; nurses are reluctant to report usually because of fear of the consequences. (p. 458)

    c.   See list, p. 458-460

24. What is the role of the nurse manager in the risk management system? How may the behavior of the nursing manager influence a risk incident?

    a.   The manager has a key role. The manager is the first line of communication and may prevent a suit. The manager also sets the tone on the unit and can help prevent litigation resulting from incidents.

    b.   See areas on key behaviors for handling complaints(p. 462), documentation (p. 462), attitude (p. 462) and analysis (p.463).

CHAPTER 22 - DEALING WITH CONFLICT

TRUE/FALSE:

1. Conflict is detrimental to any organization; it should be eliminated as quickly as possible.

2. Disruptive conflict places an emphasis on winning while competitive conflict emphasizes defeating the opponent.

3. Conflict results from different goals, values and beliefs, competition for scarce resources, group processes and task interdependencies.

4. While there are many ways to deal with conflict, five of the more common styles are the avoider, the friendly helper, the compromiser, the tough battler and the problem solver.

5. Conflict is inevitable. Many times the nurse manager will have to intervene in a conflict if the parties involved cannot settle the matter independently. When this occurs, mediation can often be used to resolve the conflict.

Answers:

1. False, p. 467
2. False, p. 468
3. True, p. 469
4. True, pp. 474-475
5. True, pp. 479-480

MULTIPLE CHOICE:

6. The presence of conflict: (p. 467)

   * a. is inevitable in all organizations
   b. reflects the occurrence of a negative process in the organization
   c. consistently leads to destructive results
   d. indicates poor managerial skills

7. Conflict can be viewed as well-managed if it achieves all of the following except: (p. 479-481)

   a. stimulation of competition
   b. increased motivation
   c. increased employee trust
   * d. lowered productivity

8. Which of the following would contribute to increased conflict in a health care institution? (pp. 469-472)

   a. increased complexity of delivering health care
   b. the changing role of professional nurses

c.   competition between health care institutions
d.   governmental regulations decreasing the length of stay
*   e.   all of the above

9. Conflict is positive when it leads to all of the following except:
    (p. 467)

    a.   increased sensitivity of problems
    b.   development of new facts
    c.   discovery of novel solutions
    d.   awareness of costs and benefits of services
*   e.   win-lose competition

10. Which of the following would be most likely to lead to conflict?
     (p. 469-472)

     a.   similar goals between departments
     b.   compatible values and attitudes between groups
*   c   scarce resources
     d.   multiple departmental goals

11. Intragroup conflict will be most likely to occur in which of the
     following situations? (p. 473)

     a.   when group membership is stable
     b.   when group values are similar among members
*   c.   when group norms are violated
     d.   when group members share similar tasks

Situation 1

Mrs. Jones has just been admitted by wheelchair to the oncology nursing unit.
Ms. White, transport aide from radiology, arrives at Mrs. Jones' room with a
wheelchair just as Ms. Smith, R.N. is completing Mrs. Jones' admission
history. The transport aide states "I'm supposed to take Mrs. Jones for her
chest x-ray." Mrs. Jones responds, "I can't do that now. I'm too worn out.
Just let me rest." Ms. White comments, "They're going to be angry with me."

12. The most important antecedent condition to conflict in this situation is:
     (p. 470)

     a.   task interdependency
*   b.   incompatible goals
     c.   difference in values
     d.   scarce resources

13. Ms. Smith's best response as problem-solver in resolving this conflict
     is: (p. 477-479)

     a.   to tell Mrs. Jones that the x-ray won't take long and that she
          can rest when she returns
     b.   to ask Ms. White to return in 30 minutes
     c.   to tell Ms. White to explain to the x-ray department that Mrs.

165

Jones will need another time for her x-ray
* d. to encourage Mrs. Jones to rest and to tell Ms. White that she will call and explain the situation to the x-ray department

Situation 2

Ms. Smith recalls other situations in which patients have been transported to the x-ray department at a scheduled time, but were required to wait for long periods of time. Other patients have reported feeling weak after their x-rays while waiting to be returned to their rooms.

14. Ms. Smith discusses her concerns with her nurse manager. The nurse manager should first: (p. 479-480)

    a. act as mediator between Ms. Smith and the radiologist
* b. decide if, when, where, and how to intervene
    c. confront x-ray staff when a problem develops
    d. schedule a meeting in the radiologist's office

15. The problem solving technique that is most likely to promote the nurse manager's success in resolving conflict in this situation if the nurse manager meets with the head of the radiology department is: (p. 475)

    a. negotiation
    b. compromise
    c. authority
* d. collaboration
    e. smoothing

16. When the individual feels that expectations conveyed by someone else are conflicting or contradictory, this problem is called: (p. 474)

    a. intra-role conflict
* b. intra-sender conflict
    c. inter-role conflict
    d. person-role conflict

ESSAY QUESTIONS

17. What is the difference between managing conflict and preventing it? Is one or the other a sounder approach? Explain.

> There is a difference. Preventing conflict involves taking actions to prevent any conflict between groups (functional or dysfunctional) from occurring. Managing conflict involves allowing conflict to exist if it is functional and taking actions to prevent its transformation to dysfunctional conflict. Managing conflict is the sounder approach because if all conflict is prohibited, organizations will become stagnant and unable to deal with change. (p. 474)

18. Are there circumstances when a manager might deliberately introduce conflict into a group?

Yes. Conflict is often introduced to reinvigorate the perspectives and energy of the group by introducing into the group an outsider ("new blood") with different perspectives, background and attitudes from group members. Conflict is also introduced to spur competition between groups. (p.476)

19. How might you apply some of the conflict management strategies from this chapter to improving union-management relations during contract negotiations?

Problem solving and compromise are two techniques that can be used to directly reach agreement on a contract. In the context of one of these strategies, smoothing can be used to emphasize the parties' common interests and, if one exists, a common enemy can be identified (e.g., a competitor that threatens the company's survival) to remind the parties that their superordinate goal is organizational survival which is only possible with the combined efforts of management and employees. (p. 476-481)

20. What is conflict? Using Filley's model of conflict resolution, describe the conflict process specific to the nurse manager. What are antecedent conditions? What behaviors may be observed?

    a. See several definitions, p. 468.
    b. See Figure 22-1, p. 469.
    c. See causes of conflict, pp. 469, 471.
    d. See manifest behavior, p. 472.

21. As organizations grow in size and complexity, interdependence increases, goal differences grow, and work and people become specialized. Does this suggest conflict in organizations must increase? Does knowledge of these changes help us prepare for them? How? (p. 471)

Usually conflict does increase with organizational growth because the number and specialization of groups in organizations increase, and the differences in perspectives, perceptions, and goals across the groups increases. (p. 524)

22. How may conflict be managed? Discuss both effective and ineffective modes of response. Identify and describe the three types of conflict outcomes and their respective strategies. Identify a situation where each respective strategy would be advantageous for the nursing manager.

    a & b. see lists, p. 474-476
          avoid, smooth, force, compete, negotiate, collaborate, compromise, confront
    c. win-lose, lose-lose, win-win (p. 476)
    d. open question, see p. 476-479

23. Describe the conflict intervention process. When should intervention be avoided?

a. see list p. 475, personal styles of intervention on p. 474, and other technique on p. 478
b. when the parties are likely to solve the problem themselves without harm to the institution (p. 480)

24. What rules should the nurse manager follow when acting as a mediator? Why are these rules important?

    a. See list, p. 480
    b. Mediation is very difficult, anything that helps the nurse manager do it is important

25. Describe conflict resolution and conflict suppression.

    See previous Questions 1, 3, and 6

26. How do factors such as role conflict and intra-professional divisiveness lead to conflict for nurses? What other factors influence conflict in nursing?

    This is an open question.

CHAPTER 23 - POWER AND POLITICS

TRUE/FALSE:

1. The politics of patient care and nursing management may cause frustration for the nurse, but have no effect on the quality of patient care.

2. Many nursing organizations, such as the American Nurses Association, its constituent state nurses organizations, the National League for Nursing, and specialty nursing organizations, influence governmental legislation and regulations.

3. Nurses can develop a positive image of power by presenting themselves as caring and compassionate experts.

4. Physicians and hospital administrators are the best prepared providers to understand the needs and wants of clients.

5. Licensure and professional regulation are the responsibility of the federal government.

Answers:

    1. False,   p. 484
    2. True,   p. 486
    3. True,   p. 489-491
    4. False,   p. 492
    5. False,   p. 493

MULTIPLE CHOICE:

6. Politics may involve influencing (p. 487)

        a. money
        b. nurses' time
        c. personnel
        d. material resources
    *   e. all of the above

7. All of the following are true about politics except: (p. 487)

        a. politics is a means to an end
        b. politics is an interpersonal endeavor
        c. politics is a collective endeavor
    *   d. politics are unnecessary in nurses' everyday work

8. The politically astute nurse will: (p. 487)

        a. avoid crossing hierarchical lines
    *   b. develop a wide support base
        c. not need knowledge of the organizational structure
        d. serve as originator and introducer of proposed changes

9. Which of the following is least important for the nurse who is attempting to develop an image of power? (p. 488)

      a. trust of others
      b. having others identify positively with her
      c. creating confidence in the ability to make change
*   d. introduction of rapid changes without trial or test

10. The nurse manager recognizes and tells one of the staff nurses that the staff nurse has been very effective in dealing with the anxious family of one of her patients. This recognition is an example of: (p. 490 and chapter 19)

      a. coercive power
      b. referent power
*   c. reward power
      d. informational power

11. One of the staff nurses has often failed to attend educational offerings available to the staff. The nurse manager who implies that the staff nurse's evaluation will be negative is using: (p. 490 and Chapter 19)

      a. referent power
*   b. coercive power
      c. informational power
      d. reward power

12. If the only information shared with a staff member is that which others want made public, it suggests that the staff member: (p. 489)

      a. is a reliable confidant
      b. has informational power
*   c. may be involved in gossiping
      d. has referent power

13. Legitimate power is: (p. 490 and Chapter 19)

      a. based on personal influence
      b. derived from superior knowledge
*   c. associated with organizational position
      d. based on sharing valuable information

14. Women and nurses tend to be more comfortable with: (p. 490)

*   a   power-sharing
      b. power grabbing
      c. power for self-interests
      d. power for personal use

15. Individual nurses can promote an image of power by all of the following except: (p. 490-491)

*   a. addressing others by title, but using one's first name

b. initiating handshakes
c. using eye contact
d. appropriately introducing self

16. Which of the following have been found to be more favorably regarded by the American public: (p. 491)

      a. physicians
      b. hospital administrators
* c. nurses

17. From a marketing perspective, nursing's goal is to: (p. 491)

      a. communicate what nursing is going to do
      b. communicate clearly what nursing is
      c. communicate what nursing does
* d. all of the above

18. The politics of bedside care for the staff nurse involves: (p. 492)

      a. joining nursing associations
* b. influencing allocation of scarce resources
      c. lobbying in the political arena
      d. building outside coalitions with political groups

19. Developing political skills can be facilitated by all of the following except: (p. 492)

      a. serving on a policy making body
      b. participation in passing motions at a business meeting
      c. understanding formal and informal political processes
* d. all of the above

20. The first step in being able to influence governmental policies is: (p. 493)

      a. establish rapport with elected officials
* b. identifying policymakers
      c. visiting elected officials
      d. participating in a campaign

ESSAY QUESTIONS:

21. What effects on health care may result if nurses fail to be involved in the politics of nursing and health care?

      poor quality of care
      frustration and turnover of nurses
      effective utilization of nurses
      lack of available care for special groups (see p. 484-487)

22. Describe the skills that are involved in politics as a personal endeavor.

   communication
   persuasion (see p. 487)

23. How can the assessment process be used in political analysis? What components should be included?

   assessment of structure and function (see p. 488)

24. What is the function of persuasion in the planning component of the political process?

   See p. 487-489.

25. Compare the eight types of power.

   See Chapter 19.

26. Describe how community support for quality nursing and health care can be promoted. (p. 495)

   legislation
   financial support
   volunteer effort
   mobilization of public opinion
   analysis of informal power structures
   community organization

CHAPTER 24 - A PRAGMATIC VIEW OF NURSING MANAGEMENT

TRUE/FALSE:

1. Most newly graduated nurses of today are well prepared to assume managerial positions in an organization.

2. The terms career and job are synonymous.

3. A mentor is a wise and experienced person who guides, supports, and nurtures a less experienced person.

4. Nurse managers must identify with management in order to carry out organizational goals on their unit.

5. It is essential that nurse managers strive to keep up with societal, nursing and health care trends in order to be effective.

6. Nurse managers are critical in setting a positive tone that fosters mutual respect among nurses and physicians on their units.

Answers:

1. False, p. 499
2. False, p. 501
3. True, p. 504
4. True, p. 501
5. True, p. 503
6. True, p. 504

MULTIPLE CHOICE:

8. Most baccalaureate nursing programs: (p. 499)

   * a. focus on clinical nursing
     b. include indepth management courses
     c. use professional management faculties to teach management
     d. prepare well educated nurse managers

9. Which of the following statements best defines a career versus a job? (p. 501)

   * a. lifelong work characterized by commitment, personal growth, and increasing levels of responsibility
     b. careers are the same as jobs
     c. pay for hours worked

10. Nurse managers should be aware of trends in which of the following major areas? (p. 503)

    * a. social, health care, and nursing
      b. government and politics
      c. medicine, physical therapy, and pharmacy

11. Which statement least describes politics? (p. 502)

*   a.   implies immoral and unethical behavior
    b.   includes the way things are done in an organization
    c.   implies what is and what is not acceptable within the
         organization

12. Which statement least describes the role of a mentor? (p. 505-506)

     a.   Mentors give support
     b.   Mentors are the same sex as the protege and 8 to 15 years older.
     c.   Mentors are knowledgeable individuals who are willing to share
          their experiences.
*   d.   Mentors are often threatened by the protege's potential for
          equaling or surpassing them

Situation 1

You are a new manager who is spending your first day on the job. Although you
are an experienced nurse manager, you have never worked in this particular
hospital and therefore are not sure what is expected. You also do not know
any of the staff.

13. Which activity would you not set as your priority on your first workday?
     (p. 509)

     a.   meet the staff
     b.   set up your office for work
     c.   start to list your goals for the organization
     d.   begin to mark meeting dates and deadlines on your calendar
*   e.   decorate your office to communicate your personality

14. When meeting and communicating with staff, which activity would not be in
     your best interest? (p. 509)

*   a.   be unconcerned about learning names of key persons this early
     b.   meet as many people as possible on a one to one basis, starting
          with key staff
     c.   take corrective action if staff starts taking advantage of you
     d.   begin establishing informal grapevines

15. Which of the following best describes a sponsor? (p. 506)

     a.   present oriented rather than future oriented
     b.   tells one what they need to do to prepare for a leadership role,
          career advancement, and success
     c.   makes sure you know people who have influence
     d.   all of the above
*   e.   B and C

16. In order to survive in the world of nursing management, which of the
     following characteristics would you avoid? (p. 507-508)

     a.   a well developed sense of self-awareness

    b. the ability to manage work, personal and family life
*   c. interpersonal insensitivity
    d. the courage to take risks
    e. a great curiosity

17. Which of the following guidelines would a nurse manager not use when attempting to influence "the boss"? (Figure 24-3, p. 512)

*   a. capitalize on the boss's weaknesses
    b. build a strong case for what you need
    c. anticipate resistance
    d. separate need from "nice to have"
    e. be persistent

18. In today's competitive market place for hospitals, it is necessary for nurse managers to view physicians as: (p. 513)

    a. role models
*   b. nursing service customers
    c. the bosses
    d. father figures

ESSAY QUESTIONS:

19. Discuss the role of a mentor. How does this compare with the role of a sponsor? Discuss the rules for the mentor or sponsor relationship.

    a. Mentors give support, teach, tell you what to do and what you need to know. (p. 505)
    b. Sponsors are future-orientated; they "open doors" for you, they tell you what you need to do. (p. 506)
    c. See list, p. 506

20. How can a nurse manager become effective in politics?

    See p. 502 for brief discussion; also Chapter 23

21. Identify several of the key behaviors for successful nursing management. If you are a nursing manager, critique your performance using these key behaviors or critique a nursing manager with whom you are familiar.

    See list, pp. 507-508. This is an open question.

22. Is being a nurse manager a career or a job?

    This is an open question, see p. 501.

23. What types of magazines and journals should a nurse manager read in order to keep current in social, nursing and health care trends?

    See p. 503 for some examples. This is an open question.

24. Discuss the author's suggestions for leading group discussions.

    See list, p. 507.

25. Discuss the first week on the job as a nurse manager. What should you do and not do?

    See lists, p. 508-510.

S E C T I O N III

◊

EXERCISE INSTRUCTIONS FOR
THE STUDENT WORKBOOK

MODULE I: 1

Exercise: Organizational Structure and Communication Networks

Objectives:

1. To facilitate understanding of how organizational structure/communication networks affect task performance, problem solving, member satisfaction, and involvement in decision making.

2. To demonstrate the strengths/weaknesses of five types of communication networks in solving both a complex and a simple nurse management task.

3. To promote discussion of organizational concepts, e.g., horizontal versus vertical dimensions, information processing model, decentralization.

Instructor's Role: To give directions, record observations, and especially to facilitate group discussion.

Operating Procedures, Hints, and Cautions

1. Be familiar with open systems and information processing models for organizations, including such concepts as centralization, systems, horizontal, vertical, and lateral relationships, power, and congruency.

2. Make certain that all participants understand the rules of the exercise by giving specific examples.

3. Assign remaining participants to observer roles for particular groups. Ask the observers to record incidents of interest and to share their records with the large group in discussion.

4. Allow 20 to 40 minutes for discussion, for reporting on experiences, for responding to Discussion Questions, and for integrating organizational concepts.

Alternatives and Variations:

1. To reduce the time needed for the exercise, place an arbitrary time limit for completion of each task. It is likely that several groups will not finish; however, this can be noted and used as a point for discussion.

2. Do not reduce the time for discussion. Organize it by giving Group Members A from each network an opportunity to summarize the group experiences. Expand the discussion to include the differences between groups.

3.   If enough chairs are not available, place a single sheet of paper on the floor in front of every assigned chair to designate the empty office chair. Then group members can move to the sheets of paper, as if in an office.

Concluding Points:

This exercise has several implications for nurse managers that should be stressed. They are as follows:

1.   Managers have much control over the informal networks that they use to solve problems and some control over the design of the formal networks.

2.   Understanding networks can help a nurse manager design them to accomplish specific tasks.

3.   All networks involve trade-offs; e.g., one network may be more efficient, but also more costly.

4.   Nurse managers should carefully assign employees to positions in networks in order to fit those with leadership skills to leadership positions.

Reading for Preparation:

Draft, R.L. and Steers, R.M. (1986) Organizations, Glenview, IL: Scott Foresman.
Katz, D. and Kahn, R. (1978) The Social Psychology of Organizations, (2nd ed.) New York: John Wiley & Sons.
Leavitt, H.J. (1951) Some effects of certain communication patterns on group performance. Journal of Abnormal and Social Psychology, 46, 38-50
Rowland, H.S. and Rowland, B.L. (1980) Nursing Administration Handbook. Germantown, MD: Aspen.
Thayer, L. (1968) Communication and Communication Systems. Homewood, IL: Irwin.

MODULE I: 2

Exercise: Accountability Issues: Legal and Ethical Cases

Objectives:

1. To increase awareness of ethical analysis.
2. To practice making ethical/legal decisions.
3. To develop decision making strategies in ethical situations.

Instructor's Role: To facilitate group discussion of case.

Operating Procedures, Hints, and Cautions:

1. Do not assign more than two cases per class period.

2. Familiarize yourself with the codes of ethics and ethics decision analysis.

3. Read the case, discussion questions, and answers before class. Formulate your own answers.

4. Discussion question responses follow below.

Case 1 Discussion Questions

Although Diane withheld certain information, we would not characterize her conduct as deceptive. Insofar as we assume that Mr. Coughlin had chosen not to exercise his right to know more about the side effects of chemotherapy, Diane was under no obligation to tell him more. To have done so in this case would have been to confuse a right to be informed with an obligation to be informed.

As nurses and doctors rightfully move away from a norm of paternalistic deception, they must be careful not to embrace a norm of paternalistic honesty. If patients clearly indicate that they do not want to know more about their illness or treatment, it is not up to the health care professionals to make stronger persons of them or to bring them up to some ideal of informed awareness. Here, as elsewhere, genuine respect for persons requires sensitivity to individual personal differences.

Case 2 Discussion Questions

Fran, a graduate almost three decades ago from a major university school of nursing, was inclined to act in conflicting ways. One way was influenced by the historical legacy of the nursing profession, which inculcated a deferential role, and the other by her recognition of the expanded scope of contemporary professional nursing. She saw the importance of being assertive and acting upon her assessment; yet, she held back. She chose not to attempt

180

to instruct mastectomy patients until she herself talked with the surgeons which, with one particular woman, would probably not occur until after the woman had left the hospital. She hopes, of course, to obtain their approval of her plans for teaching; however, her hopes are probably unrealistic since these physicians have allowed no other nurses to instruct their patients. In attempting to define the problem, Fran asked only one question: "Should I approach the physicians with my questions?" An underlying question, which she did not explicitly identify, was, "If the physicians say that they do not want me or any other nurse or student nurse to teach their patients, should I proceed to teach without their approval or against their wishes?" By focusing attention on the first question, Fran may ignore ethical inquiry into the underlying question of whether nurses should be obedient to physicians.

Case 3 Discussion Questions

How did Valerie know not to accept the physician's orders? Perhaps she reasoned that if nurses believe that they have a moral and legal obligation to meet a client's needs, then they must take risks, both by refusing to defer to a physician whose actions impede the delivery of adequate help and by taking independent emergency action. It is within the scope of most nursing practice acts that the nurse is responsible for his/her own actions and court decisions have also charged the nurse with protecting the patient from the physician if the latter is unsafe.

The physician's decision against the IV infusion differed so radically from usual emergency treatment that the other physicians in the hospital agreed that Valerie, but not the physician, had acted more appropriately. Moreover, since Valerie's action was justified on well-grounded medical and ethical considerations, she had no reason to defend her conduct simply by an appeal to conscience. A nurse may sometimes be in a situation, however, where what a physician does falls within acceptable medical practice and the nurse can justify a refusal to carry out an order or to participate in a procedure only on the basis of conscience.

Case 4 Discussion Questions

This case raises the following questions: "What are the obligations of being a member of the nursing profession? Do these obligations include attending meetings on one's own time and expense? Working overtime?"

The American Nurses Association Code for Nurses addresses the question of responsibility to the profession. Item 8 of the Code, which states that "the nurse participates in the profession's efforts to implement and improve standards of nursing," includes an interpretive statement that "the nurse has the responsibility to monitor these ANA standards for nursing practice, service, and education in everyday practice and through voluntary participation in the profession's ongoing efforts to implement and improve standards at the national, state, and local levels." Item 11, which states that "the nurse collaborates with members of the health professions and other citizens in promoting community and national efforts to meet the health needs of the public," includes an interpretive statement that "the nurse should

181

<u>actively</u> <u>seek</u> <u>to</u> <u>promote</u> <u>collaboration</u> (emphasis ours) needed for ensuring the quality of health services to all persons." The Code clearly expresses the view that nurses have obligations not only to themselves and to clients, but to the nursing profession as well. While not stating that participation in activities to improve nursing as a discipline may require extra working hours, the Code implies as much.

Very few nurses have established independent nursing practices; rather, agencies, (e.g., hospitals, nursing homes, community health departments, schools, industries, physicians, health maintenance organizations), employ the vast majority of nurses. A nurse makes a contract with an agency in order to carry out a primary obligation to the client for the provision of safe, effective, responsible nursing, be it in the words of the ANA Code "the promotion of health, the prevention of illness," or "the alleviation of suffering." An employment contract, either written or oral, specifies a nurse's obligations in terms of working hours and specific responsibilities, as well as an agency's obligations in terms of pay, benefits, vacations, etc. In addition, nurses often feel obligated to do more than the contract specifies because they fall into the "compassion trap" by accepting the expectations of many agency employers, health care workers, and clients that nurses, as members of a "helping profession," will subordinate their own needs or desires to those of others.

To return to the nurses in the case, both Diane and Arlene share high ideals about professionalism, and as dedicated nurses, both are also affected by the "compassion trap" with its assumption that the nurse will sacrifice for others. Therefore, Diane is somewhat discouraged by Arlene's recent comments about only working for pay. Peggy Sayre, another nurse from a different unit in the hospital and a friend of both women, suggested that Diane, Arlene, and she talk during a break about problems relating to Diane's working extra. After listening to the other two nurses describe the situation, Peggy asked each of them why they felt as they did about working extra.

Diane had no difficulty in pointing out that her involvement with the interdisciplinary team and working on hospital procedures would lead to better care for a larger number of clients. She also emphasized that her professional goals of high-quality nursing care and the hospital's current inclusion of her in the multidisciplinary team were in perfect agreement.

Arlene acknowledged that Diane's contributions to client welfare were admirable but quickly shifted to her own feelings concerning Diane's extra work. Arlene believes that because Diane functioned as a "supernurse" the nurse manager looked upon Arlene and several other nurses who could not devote extra time to hospital matters as less than adequate professional nurses. Furthermore, they themselves were beginning to feel inadequate. One way for them to restore their private as well as professional self-esteem would be for them to match Diane's work load by working extra hours. Arlene predicted that client welfare would be negatively affected, however, since she and most of the other nurses would be worn out by the combination of home duties, regular job, and extra unpaid work.

Arlene also said that, perhaps more importantly, she believes the way a nurse feels about him/herself as a professional affects the way in which

182

he/she approaches nursing care. Although Arlene did not think that her
negative feelings about her current level of participation in nursing matters
at the hospital had affected her practice, she thought that if her morale
continued to deteriorate, her nursing might suffer. She also predicted that
if the nurses continued to see themselves as inadequate even though they did
their best during every working hour, some of them would quit. The resulting
nursing personnel turnover would cause confusion and a reduction of the high-
quality nursing care now being provided. Furthermore, Arlene believes that if
a high turnover rate persisted, the "good" that Diane's extra work did would
be undermined.

Peggy thought that both Diane and Arlene had missed the major issue. As
for Arlene, Peggy did not believe that the decline in unit morale and the
increase in nursing staff turnover would be as great as Arlene predicted, but
she agreed that these were important concerns. More importantly, she believed
that Arlene, who recognized that she must meet her basic duties as a nurse and
honor her contract with the hospital, had not completely accepted the view
that idealized commitments to professional nursing might be overriden by other
more stringent and immediate commitments such as those to her children.
Arlene, like all nurses, had personal as well as professional obligations; and
as a single parent, she did not need to apologize for not working more than a
40-hour week. Peggy illustrated her point by describing a public health
nurse, whom they all know, who had been extremely active in collective-
bargaining activities in the county health department. When her mother had
become seriously ill and needed her every evening, the nurse could no longer
attend special nightly meetings. Her obligations to her sick parent, while
not excusing her from her contractual obligations to the health department,
did excuse her from the additional commitments she had previously taken on.
Arlene's personal obligations, like those of the public health nurse, were
more basic and thus took precedence over her less stringent professional
obligations.

Neither was Peggy convinced by Diane's argument that her professional
nursing goals were being met, and that the end result would be an overall
improvement in client welfare. Although she agreed with Diane that the
initiation of a new program or change often required an initial period of
voluntary effort, she argued that as soon as the program's value was
recognized, it was necessary to press for its institutionalization. In
Diane's case, Peggy believed, Diane had amply demonstrated the value of what
she was doing. Therefore, she should now take steps to make hers a paying,
institutionalized position. Peggy pointed out that since Diane's work
depended entirely upon one nurse's willingness to work extra, when she left
her current position for one with more responsibility--which all three nurses
agreed that a young, effective nurse like Diane would do within a short time--
there would probably be no one to carry on her good work. Nor, since the
hospital had gotten Diane's work free, would their employer believe that
another nurse would not also step forward to give free time and effort to the
hospital.

Peggy predicted that at Diane's departure, there would be no nursing
contribution to the multidisciplinary team or to similar activities since no
institutional changes to provide for participation by nurses would be made so
long as Diane functioned as she did. Therefore, in the long run, clients

would not be well served by nursing. Thus, Diane was not meeting her professional goals when the future was considered. Peggy summarized her position by saying that Diane's extra work was a problem because the nurses on the unit could not determine if Diane's special activities were merely an extension of the efforts to be professional by providing the highest quality nursing care possible or if she had slipped into the hospital's institutionalized system of devaluing nursing, although the system was obviously more subtle than that which nineteenth-century hospitals had used to exploit nurses. To Peggy, the major issue was that if Diane continued to attend special meetings without compensation, she would actually support the notion that her activities were not truly part of a nurse's employee role and that the hospital had no obligation to support nurses who work long hours to write procedures and participate in multidisciplinary team meetings.

To return to the questions raised by this case, a nurse has certain obligations to the nursing profession, as discussed in the ANA Code for Nurses. At times those obligations may include working overtime and attending meetings on one's own time and expense. But as this case illustrates, when a nurse critically examines his/her obligations, he/she may see that basic personal commitments sometimes override less stringent professional commitments that might be met by "working extra." He/she may also see that "working extra," while appearing to fulfill professional obligations and the ideal of compassionate service, may only superficially meet obligations to clients and may actually lead to a less desirable state of affairs not only for nursing colleagues and the nursing profession, but ultimately for clients. A better alternative for Diane's continued contribution to the profession would be for her to become active in her professional organization or in political activities, to teach health care classes in her community, or to continue her own education, either through formal course work or continuing education. The responsibility for the profession remains, but not at the expense of one member.

Case 5 Discussion Questions

As the Associate Director of Nursing, Ms. Romero's primary obligation is to provide safe, effective nursing care to all clients served by the hospital. Clients must be guaranteed that nurses will always be clearheaded and not under the influence of alcohol or mind-altering drugs. On the other hand, Ms. Romero also has a responsibility to help her employees function to the best of their ability. Thus, there was a conflict between Ms. Romero's professional obligations to patients and to colleagues.

Ms. Romero knew that Ms. Altmann would have daily access to drugs and that consequently she would face extraordinary temptations to steal drugs for her own use. Yet, she also recognized that the length of Ms. Altmann's previous nursing experience and the fact that she had not been found stealing drugs decreased the probability that drug-related problems would interfere with her effectiveness as an RN. Given these reasons, Ms. Romero thought it would be wrong simply to refuse to rehire Ms. Altmann. Therefore, Ms. Romero encouraged her to attend weekly drug treatment counseling sessions and waited until Ms. Altmann's therapist submitted a written statement that she was able to work safely in a clinical setting before employing her again. Rather than sacrificing either her professional obligations or her personal desire, Ms. Romero apparently found a solution that satisfied both. The case developed as follows:

The law says that nurses, as well as other people, may not steal drugs. Although it is understandable that Ms. Romero feels a personal loss since she sincerely wished for Ms. Altmann's success and gave her practical support, the law and hospital policy require that Ms. Romero must discharge and report Ms. Altmann in order to protect clients from possible unsafe care.

Ms. Romero could simply ignore the situation or excuse her drug use. But either of these courses would have a number of undesirable effects: (1) Ms. Romero would be violating the law and thus involving herself in possible legal difficulties; (2) she would be disregarding professional nursing standards; (3) she would be ignoring a strong sign that Ms. Altmann's future clients might be deprived of needed pain-relieving drugs; and (4) she would be contributing to Ms. Altmann's continued dependence on drugs. These possible consequences make it unacceptable for Ms. Romero either to ignore or excuse her drug use.

It is well accepted that drug dependency/alcoholism is a disease and is treatable. Just as anyone suffering from a disease, the nurse should be offered treatment rather than punishment. However, the nurse has had treatment and still relapsed. Ms. Romero could explore the possibility of inpatient treatment for Ms. Altmann, keeping her employed on a medical leave during her treatment in order to provide medical insurance benefits. That way, Ms. Romero could help her colleague and keep her patients safe.

This case suggests different approaches to the basic question of how a nurse ought to resolve a conflict between professional obligations to patients and to employees. When Ms. Altmann's situation appeared to be no clear threat to the provision of safe, effective care, Ms. Romero was able to identify a course of action that appeared to satisfy conflicting claims. At this point, the case underscored a suggestion made earlier in this chapter--that it is sometimes possible to select a course of action which allows one to reconcile what may appear to be competing alternatives.

Does the fact that this case did not proceed as expected imply that Ms. Romero's initial response was wrong? No, we think it does not. Sometimes it happens that the right decision in a particular case turns out badly.

Case 6 Discussion Questions

Alice believes that both nurses and patients would benefit from a strike. Her two main arguments for a nurses' strike appear to be that it would (1) benefit clients by producing changes which would improve the quality of nursing, and (2) benefit nurses by reducing job stress and requests that they work overtime. In an ideal situation, the nursing care that a hospital demands of its staff does not conflict with the nursing care which nurses believe they should provide. But Alice and the other nurses repeatedly find themselves in situations where they can only provide what they regard as substandard care because of the low ratio of nurses to patients. In Alice's view, the hospital's substandard health care is related to its exploitation of the nursing staff. The question now is whether a strike aimed at correcting the situation is ethically justified.

Deciding to initiate or participate in any form of work stoppage (e.g., sit downs, mass resignations, strikes) is difficult for nurses because of their education and experience as people in a service profession and their inexperience in collective bargaining. Strikes are especially problematic because they amount not only to withdrawing services, but also to using the resulting distress as leverage to coerce the hospital or agency into meeting the strikers' demands. Even if efforts are made to provide a warning and to staff certain units, such as intensive care, emergency rooms, and a minimal number of general nursing units, the strike will still force some people to wait for care, at the very least inconveniencing them and possibly even harming them. Since nursing strikes by their very nature require nurses to threaten patient services, such strikes bear a heavy burden of justification.

The presumption against nursing strikes, like the presumptions against paternalism, deception, and coercion, is very strong. Not only may strikes inconvenience and possibly harm clients, they are also likely to backfire. As with strikes by other groups providing vital social services, such as police and fire departments, the public is likely to respond negatively when striking nurses seem to be using the sick and infirm as hostages to better their position. Such public perceptions may be detrimental not only to the strikers, but also to the entire profession of nursing. Moreover, even if a nursing strike is successful, lingering acrimony between the strikers on the one hand and hospital administrators, physicians, and the public on the other may seriously compromise whatever gains the strike achieved.

Although the presumption against nursing strikes is very strong, it is not impossible to justify a nursing strike. Like the presumptions against paternalism and deception, it can, at least in principle, be overridden by appeal to certain ethical considerations.

Alternatives and Variations:

Do not skip the individual written analysis. It may be graded but need not be. This represents the student's practice: the class discussion is feedback. If you shortcut the written analysis, you shortchange the student's learning process.

The discussion may occur in groups of 5 to 10, but would be better with the whole class participating and you facilitating discussion.

Concluding Points:

1.   Do not be quick to solve the problem; let the students discuss it and defend what they have written.

Reading for Preparation:

Baum, R. (Ed.) (1976) <u>Ethical Arguments for Analysis</u>, (2nd ed.). New York: Holt, Rinehart & Winston.
Benjamin, M. and Curtis, J. (1981) <u>Ethics in Nursing</u>. New York: Oxford University Press.
Curtin, L. (1978) A proposed mode for critical ethical analysis. <u>Nursing Forum</u>, 17:12.
Fenner, K.M.(1980)<u>Ethics and Law in Nursing</u>. New York: Van Nostrand
Husted, G.L. and Husted, J. (1991) <u>Ethical Decision Making in Nursing</u>, St.Louis, Mosby.

MODULE I: 3

Exercise: Hospital Subunits Problem: Setting Up the First Hospital Station on Jupiter

Objectives:

1. To provide experience in resolving conflicts among subunits.

2. To aid in team-building skills.

3. To comprehend the complexity of systems and suboptimization.

Instructor's Role: To provide instructions and facilitate large group discussion.

Operating Procedures, Hints, and Cautions:

1. Be sure that participants do **not** read ahead for this exercise. If they do, their actions will not be spontaneous and the experience will be diminished.

2. Encourage participants to stick to time limits. Discussions can go indefinitely and time limits are realistic in a hospital setting.

3. This exercise can generate much group discussion at the end. Therefore, leave enough time to complete the questions as well as share experiences.

Alternatives and Variations:

This exercise is not easily altered by eliminating sections without losing its value for creating an understanding of subunits conflicts and their impact on organizations.

Concluding Points:

1. Because of the intensive technology in health care, subunit groups must find a way to coordinate their efforts. The primary concern is delivery of satisfactory patient care.

2. The organizational hierarchy of roles develops to coordinate and control the patient care delivery process.

Reading for Preparation:

Filley, A.C. (1975) Interpersonal Conflict Resolution. Glenview, IL:
    Scott, Foresman.
Katz, D. and Kahn, R. (1978) The Social Psychology of Organizations,
    New York: Wiley & Sons.
Rowland, H.S. and Rowland, B.L. (1985) Nursing Administration Handbook, 2nd
    Ed. Germantown, MD: Aspen.
Silber, M.B. (1984) Managing confrontations: Once more into the breach.
    Nursing Management, 15(4):54.

MODULE II: 1

Exercise: Self-Esteem and Self-Assessment: Two Critical Areas of Self-Awareness.

Objectives:

1.   To provide an assessment of self-perceptions that affect managerial success.

2.   To encourage openness in exploring oneself in order to increase development as a manager.

3.   To promote understanding of self-esteem and cognitive style.

Instructor's Role: To facilitate small and large group discussion and encourage participants to self-disclose.

Operating Procedures, Hints, and Cautions:

1.   This exercise requires participants to disclose their weaknesses to others. This is more easily done in small groups. Don't expect the spokesperson to divulge the details of the discussion, only a summary of main points.

2.   Be sure to clarify with participants any problems/questions they have about the questionnaires. Emphasize that this is for growth and that there are no right or wrong answers. The scoring key may be found below.

Scoring Key: Self-Esteem
Items 1-6 : a=1, b=2, c=3, d=4
Items 7-10: a=4, b=3, c=2, d=1

Total Score
10-19 Strong self-concept
20-25 Moderate self-concept
26-40 Self-esteem needs bolstering

Alternatives and Variations:

Omit the large group discussion if participants feel more comfortable in small groups. If you do so, be sure to summarize the major issues/points in the exercise.

Concluding Points:

1.   There is no one style that is preferable; there are individual characteristics that, once identified, can be used for self-development.

190

Reading for Preparation:

McKenney, J.L. and Keen, D.G.W. (1974) How managers' minds work. Harvard Business Review, 51, 79-90

MODULE II: 2

Exercise: Basic Survival Skills: What You Need to Be a Good Manager for the Future

Objectives:

1.   To provide an assessment of the individual's development in essential management skills.

2.   To promote an increased awareness of the need to plan a career.

3.   To aid in determining a set of goals for the individual's development as a nurse manager.

Instructor's Role: To facilitate the self-assessment and goalsetting process and monitor small group discussion.

Operating Procedures, Hints and, Cautions:

1.   Be familiar with the areas of critical management skills and leadership abilities.

2.   Encourage participants to be honest in their responses in order to make this exercise of value to them. Help participants to be open with each other regarding strengths and weaknesses. Each participant should mention both personal strengths and weaknesses.

3.   Read the exercise in the Student Workbook and be prepared to interpret the scoring for the Management Skills Questionnaire.

4.   The Career Plan Form may be most difficult for students. Discuss this briefly before starting the exercise. All students should be able to complete at least their first job plans, even if they are tentative.

5.   While participants are working on the Personal Goals Form, encourage a laboratory atmosphere such that participants help each other think of specific plans for self-improvement. You may bring along your own completed Personal Goals Form to demonstrate for them.

6.   Emphasize the need to plan a career. This is one area which many people, especially women, fail to address until it is too late.

Alternatives and Variations:

1.   If the participants seem to be having difficulty, demonstrate your own Personal Goals Form, Career Plan Form and Management Skills Questionnaire. This will greatly open up the group to self-disclosure.

2.   If the group is small (below 10), this is a good exercise to

complete as a whole group. It promotes sharing and openness as well as the opportunity to get fresh ideas from others on self-development.

Concluding Points:

1. Some of the major reasons why managers fail are as follows: their strengths become weaknesses, e.g., loyalty can become over-dependence; deficiencies become more prominent the higher they climb; success and power "go to their heads"; economic and political events shape their destinies negatively.

2. Knowing oneself intimately and having goals can help to circumvent those pitfalls.

3. Self-assessment is a continuing process. No matter how high we climb, we must continue to examine our needs, goals, and positives/negatives.

Reading for Preparation:

Boyatzis, R.E. (1982) The Competent Manager. New York: John Wiley & Sons.
Drucker, P.F. (1986) The Frontiers of Management, New York,
    Truman Talley Books.
Katz, R.L. (1974) Skills of an effective administrator. Harvard Business
    Review, 51:90.
Sayles, L. (1979) Leadership: What Effective Managers Really Do and
    How They Do It, New York: McGraw-Hill
Thompson, A.M. and Wood, M.D. (1980) Management Strategies for Women.
    New York: Simon and Schuster.

MODULE II: 3

Exercise: Nurse Manager Rights: Rehearsal and Fantasy

Objectives:

1. To facilitate acceptance of basic human rights for nurse managers.

2. To increase awareness of the inner messages that prevent nurses from accepting their rights.

3. To promote identification of the particular rights that are difficult for an individual to accept and to develop permissive messages to counteract this nonacceptance.

Instructor's Role: To lead large group discussion, monitor small group discussions, and direct dyad experiences.

Operating Procedures, Hints, and Cautions:

1. Be familiar with the role of rights in assertive communication in health care settings.

2. Encourage identification of as many limits/responsibilities as possible in Step 2 of the Procedure. This is essential to balancing the exercise and preventing unrealistic or insensitive use of the rights list.

3. Before class, read the directions for the guided fantasy with pauses, to familiarize yourself with the pace. Speak clearly but calmly to induce relaxation.

4. Students may have some difficulty thinking of permission statements. Be prepared to generate supportive, permissive statements for examples.

5. Leave enough time for discussion at the end, which is necessary for this exercise. Encourage students to think of how accepting rights affects their communications with others by allowing them to communicate openly, assertively and effectively.

Alternatives and Variations:

1. If space permits, students can stretch out on the floor, which may promote more relaxation and better fantasizing.

2. If time is constrained, reducing the number of statements in the dyad exercise can save time. Do not skimp on the discussion at the end. The instructor may also save time by eliminating the dyad or the fantasy.

<u>Concluding Points</u>:

1. All of us have difficulty accepting some rights and not others. Our inability to accept a certain right is often an outgrowth of our socialization process.

2. Practicing giving ourselves permission to have rights can increase our confidence in this area.

3. All rights carry responsibilities and if we accept the rights, we need to examine and accept the responsibilities.

<u>Reading for Preparation</u>:

Alberti, R. and Emmons, M. (1974) <u>Your Perfect Right</u>.
    San Luis Obispo: Impact Publishers.
Chenevert, M. (1978) <u>Special Techniques in Assertiveness Training for
    Women in the Health Professions</u>. St. Louis: C.V. Mosby.
Jakubowski-Spector, R. (1973) <u>An Introduction to Assertive Training
    Procedures for Women</u>. Washington D.C.: American Personnel and
    Guidance Association

195

MODULE II: 4

Exercise: Role Clarification and Authority Limits for the Nurse Manager

Objectives:

1.   To promote understanding of the complexities of the role of nurse manager.

2.   To explore this role in the organization by determining superior, subordinate, and lateral relationships.

3.   To encourage clarification of authority limits for nurse managers.

4.   To examine potential solutions to role conflict.

Instructor's Role: To provide direction and facilitate small and large group discussions.

Operating Procedures, Hints, and Cautions:

1.   Be familiar with the basic concepts in role theory and types of organizational relationships, i.e., lateral, subordinate, and superior.

2.   Be familiar with the job description for nurse management in the text and the Authority Limits and Role Questionnaires in the Student Workbook (Exercise II-4).

3.   Remember that some students will have had supervisory experience and some will not. Mixing experienced with nonexperienced students can increase the breadth of discussion in the small groups.

4.   Learning from this exercise can be enhanced by discussions of power/influence relating to organizational relationships and interdependencies among departments.

5.   Encourage students to see the role of nurse manager as complex and relationships as two-way. For example, as a nurse manager you may have authority to sign off for patients to do x-ray from your unit; however, you may have to obtain sign-off from x-ray when sending x-rays of a patient on your unit to a doctor's office.

Alternatives and Variations:

The time required for this exercise can be reduced by specifying only certain items to be discussed on the questionnaires or by eliminating the small group discussions and using the whole group for all steps in the exercise. This is not recommended for classes over 20 in size.

Concluding Points:

The following ideas for solutions to role conflicts should be discussed in class:

1.   Prioritizing your role obligations. For example, fulfilling a superior's expectations may be more important than solving a subordinate's problem at some point in time.

2.   Clarifying your relationships in the organization. For example, you can review the relationships described in the questionnaire. This will help you to identify sources of power and support in the organization.

3.   Discussing your role functions with your supervisor. Make a special effort to set a mutual understanding about your role with your supervisor.

4.   Working on self-development. Periodically review the strengths and weaknesses in your performance in your role and with the lateral relationships in the organization.

5.   Developing mentor relationships. Mentors can give you more support and more opportunities to influence your lateral and superior relationships. This will make you a more effective manager for your unit.

6.   Separating your roles. Determine the different expectations for your role as superior versus your role as subordinate or as a peer. Clearly make these distinctions.

Reading for Preparation:

Halley, W.H. and Jennings, K.M. (1983) Personnel Management: Functions and Issues, New York, Dryden Press.
Katz, D. and Kahn, R. (1978) The Social Psychology of Organizations. New York: Wiley & Sons.
Thompson, A.M. and Wood, M.D. (1980) Management Strategies for Women. New York: Simon & Schuster.

MODULE III: I

Exercise: Nonverbal Behavior in Communication

Objectives:

1. To increase awareness of the role of nonverbals in communication.

2. To provide a framework for understanding nonverbals in communicating and for interpreting nonverbal behaviors.

3. To provide practice in communicating/interpreting nonverbal cues and the opportunity for feedback regarding nonverbal communication of feelings.

Instructor's Role: To direct dyad exercises and monitor small group experience, helping leaders when needed.

Operating Procedures, Hints, and Cautions:

1. Be familiar with the research on nonverbal communication.

2. Allow 3 to 4 minutes for each of the dyad exercises a through e. Defer discussion until e is complete.

3. In the whole group discussion, focus on the concept of the "behavior paradox," i.e., that we cannot "do nothing." We are always communicating nonverbally. Include a discussion of attention and how we communicate that nonverbally, eye contact and problems with too much or too little.

4. Determine the number of small groups and prepare that number of sets of "emotion" cards. Print one on each card, i.e., love, joy, confidence, anger, bafflement, powerlessness, anxiety, and disgust. Be certain that participants do not see the cards.

5. Instruct the leader of each small group to help the members express emotions. Walk around the room and offer suggestions and encouragement. Remind participants of the role of no words.

Alternatives and Variations:

1. To reduce the time needed for the exercise, have the participants portray only two emotions. Do not reduce the discussion periods.

2. If participants have some experience with concepts in nonverbal communication, skip the dyad exercises and start with a general discussion of nonverbal communication.

Concluding Points:

Summarize the factors in interpreting nonverbal behaviors.

Reading for Preparation:

Baker, H.K. and Morgan, P., Building a Professional Image: Using Feeling-Level Communication, Supervisory Management, January, 1986, p. 20-25
Clark, C. (1977) Nonverbal Communication in Nursing Concepts & Processes. Albany, New York: Delmar.
Fast, J. (1971) Body Language, New York: Pocket Books.

MODULE III: 2

Exercise: Active Listening

Objectives:

1. To promote improved listening skills.

2. To provide the opportunity for feedback from others in active listening.

3. To teach the technique of active listening.

Instructor's Role: To facilitate dyad exercises, monitor triad role plays, and lead large group discussion.

Operating Procedures, Hints, and Cautions:

1. Be familiar with the technique of active listening.

2. Help participants to see the difference between feeling and content messages.

Alternatives and Variations:

1. Encourage participants to derive their own situations for active listening.

2. Practice several other components of active listening in dyads prior to the triad role play if participants are new to listening skills.

Concluding Points:

1. Limits must be set on listening in the workplace. Participants need to learn to handle a speaker who talks continuously or acts defensively. Explore solutions to these situations.

2. Listening requires full concentration. If you are preoccupied with other things, you can't listen well. Simply letting the speaker know this and setting another time to talk can be effective in this situation.

Reading for Preparation:

Erust, F., Jr. (1973) Who's Listening? A Handbook of the T.A. of
    the Listening Function. Vallejo, CA: Addresso set.
Morgan, P. and Baker, H.K., (Nov., 1985) Building a Professional Image;
    Improving Listening Behavior," Supervisor Management, p. 34-36

Exercise: Writing Memos Effectively

Objectives:

1. To provide practice in writing memos to communicate with staff.

2. To promote increased awareness of the importance of written communications.

Instructor's Role: To facilitate large group discussion, provide guidance, and monitor small group discussion.

Operating Procedures, Hints, and Cautions:

1. Be familiar with the writing skills that are needed in nursing.

2. In small groups, encourage participants to consider carefully the audience and voice.

3. Provide appropriate reasons for the "model" memo during the large group discussion. The model analysis and reasoning are on pages 204 to 205.

Alternatives and Variations:

Participants can bring in their completed memos and the instructor can select several from the whole group that represent a variety of styles. The group can discuss pros and cons and compare to the model. This approach will further reduce time needed for this exercise to approximately 30 minutes.

Concluding Points:

The following is a summary of items to consider in writing memos and report--the seven C's of good writing:

Clearness	Is the report understandable?
Completeness	Have all pertinent facts been given?
Conciseness	Is it precise and to the point?
Correctness	Are the facts correct?
Courtesy	Am I fair to those concerned?
Candor	Is it honest?
Character	Does it fit me?

Reading for Preparation:

Finsher, S. (July-Sept. 1985) Remark, Revise, Rewrite, Business, p. 54-55
Leggett, G. et. al. (1982) Prentice-Hall Handbook for Writers.
    (8th ed.). Englewood Cliffs, N.J.: Prentice-Hall.

Model Memo

Model Situation Analysis

Before you write, you should analyze the situation for its five key characteristics. This analysis helps you to determine exactly what you are to do. It also gives you guidelines for applying the writing skills. You should have made the following identifications:

Subject   new visiting hours for children of mothers in maternity;
             hours: 11:30 am-2 pm and 3:45 pm - 5 pm; new policy

Purpose   to inform and to explain

Audience   Nurse Managers

Form   memo--because this is an in-house communication;written-
                because this is an official policy that requires
                            documentation

Voice   clear, concise, organized, logical

Writing Preparation

Let's begin by reminding you that there is **no one correct** solution in writing situations such as this. Rather, there are different possibilities. They depend on your audience, purpose, and use of writing skills.

However, we can point out what might happen for each of the answers in our question list.

1.   Word choice is very important. With words, you will describe the new policy. If the words aren't accurate, precise, and concise, you may obscure the information. Technical terminology isn't necessary. There is no content here that needs it. You're talking about times, places, and extensions. Sentence structure is important. With it, you will create an impression of how the audience relates to change. Organization is necessary to insure logic but the arrangement can vary. Layout demands some attention but you can be flexible. Use the established hospital format for memos or use your own. Use of detail deserves attention. Select and include only what is pertinent to meet the purpose: to inform.

2.   You should choose words that are plain English and are objective. Say "visiting hours" and "children". Refer to "extension 998." Don't use words such as "sibling" and "familial encouragement visitations."

3.   Sentence tone also is important. If you use commands, you are placing your audience (other managerial professionals below you) in a "carry-out-this-order" position. So do you want to say, "Allow children to visit mothers during the 11:30 am - 2 pm and 3:45 pm - 5 pm slot"? If you say, "What do you think of allowing children to visit their mothers during the next time slots?", you don't sound sure of yourself. In fact, is the policy in effect? Try such statements as, "Beginning today, children may visit their mothers during the 11:30 am - 2 pm & 3:45 pm - 5 pm hours <u>if</u> they make an appointment the day before."

4.   If you refer to the audience as "nurse managers," you stress the professional nature of your material and relationship. If you say "staff," you sound impersonal. "To whom it may concern" is too remote.

5.   If you refer to yourself with your title, you stress professionalism. If you say "Joan," you are very informal. "J. Smith" is not complete enough for an official policy memo. Your initials "JS" may not be recognized by all. Joan Smith, RN, is an appropriate signature within your unit. Joan Smith, RN, Head Nurse, 2 South, would be appropriate within the hospital.

6.   You should arrange the material logically. There are at least two obvious logical orders: (1) source, policy, visiting hours, date, appointment; (2) date, hours, appointment, policy, source.

7.   How much detail should be included? Consider some effects. If you put in old policy and hours information, you may confuse the audience. If you include the reason for and procedure by which the old policy was changed, you may also be adding too much for this memo. It adds history to information. Conversely, staff acceptance of policy changes is critical to its success, so a few words of explanation are usually necessary.

Model Memo

Remember: there is no one right answer. But compare your memo with the one below. Note also annotations, which point out what was done and why. How does yours compare?

Blank Hospital
Any City, U.S.A.
March 3, 19--

TO: Joan Smith, RN OB Head Nurse

FROM: Gerry James, RN, Associate Director of Nursing

RE: Children's Visiting Hours

Beginning March 10, 19--, we will have a new policy and procedure for children who want to visit their mothers and new babies. They may come with an adult between

11:30 am - 2:30 pm and 3:45 pm - 5 pm

Their parents should make an appointment for the visit the morning before. They can do this by calling Ext. 998

This new policy, approved by the Department of Obstetrics and Gynecology, the Department of Nursing Services, and the Medical Board, extends our new family-centered maternity care. Encourage the patients to take advantage of it.

---

stresses	plain	includes	presents	adds
professional	English	relevant	major	secondary
relationship		detail	idea first	information

MODULE IV: 1

Exercise: Understanding Assertive, Aggressive, and Passive
         Communication

Objectives:

1.   To facilitate an understanding of the three types of
     communication, i.e., assertive, aggressive, and passive.

2.   To provide commonly encountered work situations in which to
     practice distinguishing these modes of communication.

3.   To promote identification of types of work situations in which it
     is difficult to respond assertively.

Instructor's Role: To monitor small group discussion and lead large group
discussion.

Operating Procedures, Hints, and Cautions:

1.   Be familiar with the concepts of assertive, aggressive, and
     passive behavior. Be able to clarify the differences verbally and
     nonverbally for participants.

2.   Read the exercise in the student workbook.

3.   Participants will have most difficulty distinguishing assertive
     and aggressive responses. Encourage the focus to be on nonverbal
     cues when the content is the same.

4.   Emphasize the importance of responsible assertive behavior.
     Assertiveness means concern and consideration for others, not
     unbridled put-downs and sarcasm.

5.   In the discussion questions, the focus becomes more on self-
     assessment. Clarify any points in the large group that are raised
     by the small group discussions.

Alternatives and Variations:

   Discussion questions may be addressed by the whole group. However,
   because the questions focus on self-assessment, participants may be more
   open in small groups.

Concluding Points:

1.   Assertiveness training involves understanding the concepts,
     identifying problem areas in acting assertively, reducing anxiety
     about those situations, and actively practicing new assertive
     behaviors.

2. Contrary to belief, assertiveness will not be viewed negatively by others. This is one fear that prevents many people from asserting themselves.

3. Assertiveness is one of the major qualities sought by interviewers in job interviews.

4. Fears of acting assertively can be overcome by setting up a hierarchy of fears and systematically desensitizing yourself through the use of relaxation. Another method uses cognitive restructuring to change the negative cognitions that prevent assertiveness.

Reading for Preparation:

Bower, S.A. and Bower, G.H. (1976) Asserting Yourself. Reading, MA: Addison-Wesley.

Chenevert, M. (1978) Special Techniques in Assertiveness Training for Women in the Health Professions: St. Louis: C.V. Mosby Company

Drury, S.S. (1984) Assertive Supervision, Champaign, IL., Research Press.

Herman, S. (1978), Becoming Assertive: A Guide for Nurses, New York: D. Van Nostrand Company.

Lange, A.J. and Harris, G.G. (1975) Responsible Assertive Behavior. Champaign, IL: Research Press.

Osborn, S.M. and Harris, G.G. (1975) Assertive Training for Women. Springfield, IL: Charles C. Thomas Publishing.

MODULE IV: 2

Exercise: Making and Refusing Requests

Objectives:

1. To facilitate improvements in the ability to make and refuse requests.
2. To increase awareness of the obstacles to effectively make and refuse requests.
3. To provide the opportunity for feedback from others in making/refusing requests.

Instructor's Role: To monitor dyad and triad role plays and lead a large group discussion.

Operating Procedures, Hints, and Cautions:

1. Be familiar with Exercise 1, Module IV and review the concepts of assertive, passive, and aggressive behavior.
2. Pay particular attention to ways in which participants may nonverbally discount their requests and refusals.
3. Encourage participants to give specific, constructive feedback to each other.
4. In discussions, bring out the issues of rights/responsibilities and blocks to making and refusing requests, (e.g., guilt, fear of hurting someone).

Alternatives and Variations:

1. Allow participants to make up relevant situations to be role played.
2. To reduce the time needed for this exercise, eliminate the dyad exercises, but cover the material in discussions. As an alternative, give participants the option of choosing either a request or refusal role play, based on individual need for practice.

Concluding Points:

1. There is a relationship between the abilities to make and to refuse requests. Often when a person becomes more comfortable with refusals, he/she finds it easier to make requests and vice versa. Realizing that refusals are not devastating to anyone gives a person permission to act more assertively.
2. Consider the individual and the context when making/refusing requests. Timing may make the difference between an acceptance or a refusal. Do the same for yourself when refusing, i.e., consider the time and circumstances. Don't agree to do something you don't want to do unless you have made a clear, active choice to do so based on carefully considered options.

Reading for Preparation:

Alberti, R.E. and Emmons, M.L. (1974) <u>Your Perfect Right</u>. San Luis, Obispo:
    Impact Publishers.
Smith, M.J. (1975) <u>When I Say No I Feel Guilty</u>. New York: Bantam
    Books/Dial Press

MODULE IV - 3

Exercise: Using Power and Influence

Objectives:

1. To provide knowledge of and encourage thinking about the basis of power in organizations.
2. To assess individual influence styles and practice new ways of influencing.

Instructor's Role: To lead large group discussion and monitor small group experience.

Operating Procedures, Hints, and Cautions:

1. Help students understand the dynamics of power by using relevant experiences in the discussion.
2. Encourage students to be honest about their strengths and weaknesses and to work on influence styles with which they are the least comfortable.
3. Discussion is often lively and much disagreement occurs about power. Encourage objective thinking, understanding and tolerance for different opinions.
4. Be prepared with the following explanation for the Influence Styles Assessment as follows:

There are no right or wrong answers to the questionnaire. The questionnaire measures important strategies operating in the political arena of organizational life. It is best to develop a repertoire of methods and to assess whether they are working. Your lowest score is your favored method of influencing others and your second lowest score represents your backup method. From left to right the styles are:

Reason--using facts and information to influence. This style is best used when people do not have data available. For example, when you have workflow problems and you know you need more staff. You do an analysis and submit it to the administrator.

Appeal--using loyalty, promises of recognition and future rewards. This style is emotional, can be manipulative and should not be over-used.

Involvement--using collaboration and consensus. This style does get commitment but it is often time-consuming.

Pressure--using peer pressure, threats of exposure or mobilization of key influencers. This style gets fast results but often ends in negative feelings.

Alternatives and Variations:

1. This exercise can be done in pairs if needed.
2. The instructor can provide examples of the different styles for the students or ask for their ideas about the styles and model them instead of role-playing.

Concluding Points:

1. Power is a fact of life for nurse managers in health care.
2. Becoming more comfortable with the different styles can greatly improve your effectiveness as a nurse manager.

Reading for Preparation:

Mintzberg, H. (1983) Power in and Around Organizations. Prentice Hall.
Mintzberg, H. (1989) Mintzberg on Management: Inside the Strange World of Organizations. Free Press.

MODULE V: 1

Exercise: Planning and Running a Meeting

Objectives:

1. To demonstrate a method for planning and running a meeting.
2. To provide practice in running a meeting.
3. To encourage thoughtful preparation and anticipation when using meetings.

Instructor's Role: To lead large group discussion and monitor small group experiences.

Operating Procedures, Hints, and Cautions:

1. Be familiar with group processes and steps in running a meeting.
2. Be sure that all participants have an agenda. Only one person from each group will utilize his/her agenda.
3. Strictly adhere to the "number guess" as a way to appoint a leader. Do not let participants pick leaders, as they may choose a person who needs the least practice.
4. Encourage participants to "get into" their roles.
5. Monitor the small group discussions to be sure that constructive feedback is given to the leader.
6. Be sure there is some discussion of the agenda. Is it realistic?

Alternatives and Variations:

1. If time permits, allow other group members to be leader.
2. Invent new roles and replay the scene with another leader.

Concluding Points:
1. Discuss the advantages and disadvantages to more or less group participation.
2. Discuss methods of effective speaking that are necessary to many meetings (e.g., getting the audience's attention, speaking firmly and clearly, pacing the speech, maintaining good eye contact, relating the topic to the audience, summarizing the main points).

Reading for Preparation

Gold, R.A., (1972) Are Your Meetings Like This One? Harvard Business Review, p. 68-77
Roberts, V., (1985) The Head Nurse Meeting: Who, What, When and Where, Nursing Management, p. 10-12
Thompson, A.M. and Wood, M.D. (1980) Management Strategies for Women. New York: Simon & Schuster.
Tropman, J. (1980) Effective Meetings. Beverly Hills, CA: Sage.

MODULE V: 2

Exercise: Leadership Styles: Assessment and Feedback

Objectives:

1. To promote understanding of the Ohio State leadership model.
2. To increase awareness of individual leadership style through self-assessment and group feedback.
3. To provide an experience in assessing leadership behavior in a complex group situation.
4. To apply concepts of leadership theory.

Instructor's Role: To give directions for the small group experience and to monitor small group feedback and discussion.

Operating Procedures, Hints, and Cautions:

1. Be familiar with the Ohio State Leadership model and the four leadership style quadrants.

2. Prepare a complex building toy model. It can be of any form such that it is not easily and quickly assembled by the participants. Bring enough building toys for four groups to replicate the model. Cover the model to prevent participants from viewing it. Distribute the same amount of building materials to each group.

3. Be certain the participants understand the rules of the exercise. Do not allow any written communication about the model between participants.

4. Review the questionnaires and scoring procedures carefully before class.

5. Encourage constructive feedback to the group leaders. Help participants remain nondefensive while discussing leadership strengths and weaknesses.

Alternative and Variations:

1. The time for the task can be reduced by simplifying the model; however, there will be less time for participants to rate their leaders.

2. A discussion period devoted to the questionnaire and the self-rating may be helpful in a class period following the exercise.

Concluding Points:

Discuss the application of the theory to nurse management. Nursing of the future may point to the need for a Quadrant 2 leader. Managerial styles of Quadrant 1 encourage direction with compliance, Quadrant 3 encourage security and comfort, and Quadrant 4 encourage acquiescence and resignation. Only the Quadrant 2 management style encourages open communication, mutually respecting relationships, and commitment to production, which are necessary to mature organizations such as in hospitals of today that must cope with a changing environment.

Reading for Preparation

Blake, R.R. and Mouten, J.S. (1981) Grid Approaches for Managerial Leadership in Nursing. St. Louis: C.V. Mosby Company
Filley, A.C. and House, R.J. (1969) Managerial Process and Organizational Behavior. Glenview, IL: Scott, Foresman.
Hersey, P. and Blanchard, K.H. (1972) Management of Organizational Behavior, (2nd ed.), Englewood Cliffs: Prentice-Hall.

MODULE V: 3

Exercise: Building a High Performance Team: The Zin Obelisk

Objectives:

1. To comprehend the characteristics of effective teams.

2. To provide experience in sharing information and team-problem-solving.

Instructor's Role: To provide instructions and facilitate large group discussion.

Operating Procedures, Hints, and Cautions:

1. Plan ahead for the number of groups you will have in your class. Make up the correct number of sets of Zin Obelisk Information Cards for the group (33 cards per set) typed on 3 by 5 cards (one per card). The sets of cards should be distributed randomly among the group members.

2. Allow enough time for discussion. This exercise usually generates lively discussion and sharing of experiences.

3. Be familiar with the rationale ahead of time.

Answer and Rationale:

The dimensions of the zin indicate that it contains 50,000 cubic feet of stone blocks.

The blocks are 1 cubic foot each, therefore, 50,000 blocks are required.

Each worker works 7 schlibs in a day (2 schlibs are devoted to rest).

Each worker lays 150 blocks per schlib, therefore each worker lays 1050 blocks per day.

There are 8 workers per day, therefore 8,400 blocks are laid per working day.

Since work does not take place on Daydoldrum, the sixth working day is Neptiminus.

Alternative and Variations:

Any number of groups may be directed simultaneously, as long as they each have a set of Zin Obelisk Information Cards. Extra irrelevant information may be introduced in order to complicate the task.

214

Concluding Points:

Time and experience do affect the development of a team. In the class exercise, there is not much time to develop trust, cooperation, communication and involvement.
Improving team performance is becoming more critical for health care facilities due to increasing competition.

Reading for Preparation:

Kinlaw, D. (1991) <u>Developing Superior Work Teams: Building Quality and the Competitive Edge</u>. University Associates.
Mahoney, F.X. (1981-82) Team development, <u>Personnel</u>, (seven part series).
Exercise from Francis, D. & Young, D. (1979) <u>Improving Workgroups: A Practical Manual for Team Building</u>. University Associates.

Zin Obelisk Information Cards

1.   The basic measurement of time in Atlantis is a day.
2.   An Atlantian day is divided into schlibs and ponks.
3.   The length of the zin is 50 feet.
4.   The height of the zin is 100 feet.
5.   The width of the zin is 10 feet.
6.   The zin is built of stone blocks.
7.   Each block is 1 cubic foot.
8.   Day 1 in the Atlantian week is called Aquaday.
9.   Day 2 in the Atlantian week is called Neptiminus.
10.   Day 3 in the Atlantian week is called Sharkday.
11.   Day 4 in the Atlantian week is called Mermaidday.
12.   Day 5 in the Atlantian week is called Daydoldrum.
13.   There are five days in an Atlantian week.
14.   The working day has 9 schlibs.
15.   Each worker takes rest periods during the working day totaling 16 ponks.
16.   There are 8 ponks in a schlib.
17.   Workers each lay 150 blocks per schlib.
18.   At any time when work is taking place there is a gang of 9 people on site.
19.   One member of each gang has religious duties and does not lay blocks.
20.   No work takes place on Daydoldrum.
21.   What is a cubitt?
22.   A cubitt is a cube, all sides of which measure 1 megalithic yard.
23.   There are 3 1/2 feet in a megalithic yard.
24.   Does work take place on Sunday?
25.   What is a zin?
26.   Which way up does the zin stand?
27.   The zin is made up of green blocks.
28.   Green has special religious significance on Mermaidday.
29.   Each gang includes two women.
30.   Work starts at daybreak on Aquaday.
31.   Only one gang is working on the construction of the zin.
32.   There are eight gold scales in a gold fin.
33.   Each block costs 2 gold fins.

MODULE VI: 1

Exercise: Making Decisions Rationally: Applying the Vroom and Yetton Model

Objectives:

1.   To learn a model for decision making based on rational decision rules.

2.   To help participants learn to apply the Vroom and Yetton model to management problems in nursing.

Instructor's Role: To monitor small group discussion, to organize large group discussion, and teach the model to participants.

Operating Procedures, Hints, and Cautions:

1.   Make sure that everyone understands the model before breaking into small groups.

2.   You may wish to make a transparency of the Vroom Analyses (Figure VI:1-A) for the class discussion.

3.   Encourage participants to come up with their own ideas of decision rules during the discussion.

Alternatives and Variations:

You can shorten the time needed for the exercise by doing fewer cases or doing the cases as a whole group. A poll can be taken of the various chosen decision styles among all participants.

Concluding Points:

Vroom has reported the following information from his research on over 500 managers from 11 countries and many kinds of companies:

1.   The managers' actual behavior was less variable than the behavior suggested by the model. Thus, managers need to be more flexible in their choices.

2.   The managers' actual behavior agreed with the model only 40% of the time; however, 66% of the time the managers' behavior was consistent with the feasible set.

3.   The decision rules most likely to be violated were those designed to protect the acceptance of the decision rather than the quality of the decision. Therefore, managers may be more likely to have problems with employee commitment to decisions.

4.   Managers are less likely to use participation when (a) they have all needed information, (b) the problem is well structured, (c)

subordinate acceptance is high, and (d) personal goals and organizational goals are not congruent for the employees.

Reading for Preparation:

LaMonica, E. and Finch, F. (1977) Managerial decision making. _Journal of Nursing Administration_, 7(5):20.
Vroom, V. and Yetton, D. (1973) _Leadership and Decision Making_. Pittsburgh: University of Pittsburgh.

Figure VI A
Vroom Analyses

CASE I

    Question A (Quality?)=yes
    Question B (Manager's Information?)=no
    Question C (Structured?)=no
    Question D (Acceptance?)=yes
    Question E (Prior Probability of Acceptance?)=no
    Question F (Goal Congruence?)=no
    Question G (Conflict?)=n/a

    Problem Type 13
    Feasible Set C11

CASE II

    Question A (Quality?)=yes
    Question B (Manager's Information?)=no
    Question C (Structured?)=no
    Question D (Acceptance?)=yes
    Question E (Prior Probability of Acceptance?)=no
    Question F (Goal Congruence?)=yes
    Question G (Conflict?)=n/a

    Problem Type 12
    Feasible Set G2

CASE III

    Question A (Quality?)=yes
    Question B (Manager's Information?)=no
    Question C (Structured?)=yes
    Question D (Acceptance?)=no
    Question E (Prior Probability of Acceptance?)=n/a
    Question F (Goal Congruence?)=n/a
    Question G (Conflict?)=n/a

    Problem Type 10
    Feasible Set A11

MODULE VI: 2

Exercise: Problem Solving Strategies

Objectives:

1. To teach the process of force field analysis for problem solving.

2. To increase awareness of one's needs.

3. To promote analysis of problems via a force field approach.

Instructor's Role: To monitor small group experience and provide guidance in problem analysis for each participant.

Operating Procedures, Hints, and Cautions:

1. It may be useful to complete the exercise for yourself in order to assist the class.

2. Be prepared for lively discussion. This exercise tends to inspire much involvement.

3. Encourage participants to focus on real problems in their lives. Remember that the more trust and contact among group members, the more useful this exercise will be to them.

Alternatives and Variations:

1. Have the class complete all work sheets in class, but be prepared to take two class periods to complete the exercise. You will be able to help participants more if done in this manner.

2. Share your completed work sheets with the class. This can be done most effectively if the class is smaller in size.

Concluding Points:

Discuss the following conceptual blocks to problem solving with the class:

1. Using only one thinking mode, e.g., thinking only in words rather than emotionally, visually, or symbolically.

2. Stereotyping situations based on past situations that are similar to current ones.

3. Thinking vertically only, i.e., starting with a single definition and pursuing the problem based only on that definition.

4. Defining the boundaries of problems too narrowly--not looking more broadly.

5. Failing to see the relationship between different elements, i.e., not seeing the commonalities.

6. Failing to inquire enough.

7. Tending to act before adequate time for thinking has passed.

8. Not deleting irrelevant information.

<u>Reading for Preparation</u>:

Denton, D.K., (1986) Problem Solving by Keeping in Touch, <u>Business</u>, p. 40-42.
Huber, G.P. (1980) <u>Managerial Decision Making</u>. Glenview, IL: Scott, Foresman.
Janis, I.L. and Mann, L. (1977) <u>Decision Making</u>. New York: Free Press.
Steele, S.M. and Maraviglia, M.S. (1981) <u>Creativity in Nursing</u>. Thorofare, N.J.: C.B. Slack.

MODULE VI: 3

Exercise: Decisions by Consensus, Authority, and Committee

Objectives:

1. To promote understanding of three types of decision making.

2. To increase awareness of the effects of decision-making styles on group members.

Instructor's Role: To facilitate small group experience and lead large group discussion.

Operating Procedures, Hints, and Cautions:

1. Become familiar with Vroom and Yetton's model found in Module VI: Exercise 1, and be sure that participants are too. They do not need indepth experience with the model but should understand the basics.

2. Assign a leader role to someone in the group whom you think will lead without being overly aggressive. You want the group who uses authority as a decision-making method to finish first.

3. Think over the ranking form before class and decide how you want the spokesperson to report to you. Group averages are fine, but you must allow time to figure them. This will be more difficult with larger groups.

4. In general, if groups are much larger than 30, it becomes more difficult to figure the rankings or make decisions.

Alternatives and Variations:

To reduce the time needed for the exercise, establish a time limit for the decision making process. Remember that this will be no problem for the authority group but difficult for the consensus group.

Concluding Points:

1. The nature of the situation greatly affects the choice of decision style.

2. Committees can be more cumbersome than helpful, depending upon how they are instituted.

3. Consensus decisions are often inappropriate or too time-consuming in day-to-day nurse management decisions.

Reading for Preparation:
Huber, G.P. (1980) <u>Managerial Decision Making</u>. Glenview, IL: Scott, Foresman.
Janis, I.L. and Mann, L. (1977) <u>Decision Making</u>. New York: Free Press
Steele, S.M. and Maraviglia, M.S. (1981) <u>Creativity in Nursing</u>.
   Thorofare, N.J.: C.B. Slack

<u>Scoring Procedure:</u>

The ranking according to Dr. Irwin is:

_3_	Alcohol	_6_	Heroin
_5_	Barbiturates	_7_	LSD-25
_4_	Tobacco (cigarette smoking	_8_	Marijuana
_1_	Glue sniffing	_2_	Methamphetamine

Enter these scores in column 3 on the chart and complete the last two columns.
Compare your individual total difference with that of the group.

<u>Dr. Irwin's Rationale:</u>

   <u>Glue sniffing</u> was rated highest because it leads to rapid loss of
control and consciousness, possible overdosage, and death from respiratory
arrest. It can also produce irreversible damage to the brain and bodily
tissues.

   <u>Methamphetamine</u> (or "speed"), especially when taken intravenously, was
rated second because of its high psychological dependence risk (it is too
pleasurable). It also predictably produces a paranoid schizophrenic state
with greatly impaired judgment, excitement, and a tendency for violence after
repeated use of doses three or more times what a physician might prescribe.
Taking the drug by injection leads to further impairment of functioning, a
possibility of hepatitis, septicemia and AIDS from the use of unsterile
materials, and a probable need for protective hospitalization.

   <u>Alcohol</u> was ranked third because it has a high potential for
psychological dependence in addition to physical dependence, greatly impairs
judgment and coordination (a leading cause of driving accidents), increases
aggressiveness and violent behavior, often produces marked social
deterioration, and causes irreversible damage to the brain, liver, and other
body tissues. The withdrawal symptoms (delirium tremens) from alcohol abuse
are also often life-threatening and difficult to treat.

   <u>Tobacco</u> (cigarette smoking) is listed next (fourth) because of the high
incidence of irreversible damage (to lungs, heart, and blood vessels) and
cancer formation accompanying its prolonged use. These hazards greatly reduce
the life span and often debilitate the individual long before death.

   <u>Barbiturates</u> were ranked fifth because, although similar to alcohol in
their overall effects and dependence liabilities, they do not cause as much
extensive tissue damage.

   <u>Heroin</u> was rated sixth because, unlike alcohol and barbiturates, it does
not impair coordination and judgment in normal doses, does not produce

extensive tissue damage, and is more likely to inhibit aggressive behavior. When taken intravenously, it is potentially very addictive, both psychologically and physically, and continued use can lead to social deterioration. But the physical dependence would be of relatively little consequence if the drug were available. Sufficient tolerance develops to the depressant effects so that it is possible to function more productively under the influence of heroin than with alcohol or barbiturates. The main danger from heroin (or morphine) is acute respiratory failure and death from overdose among inexperienced users, as a very narrow margin exists between the effective dose and the lethal dose. With illicit supplies varying greatly in potency, this is a serious danger. Because unsterile materials are often used for injection, there is also a risk of hepatitis, septicemia and AIDS.

LSD-25 is seventh on the list because, although it can cause psychotic reactions, such occurrences are relatively rare (less than 1 percent of volunteers in clinical settings have prolonged adverse reactions and the rate of psychotic reactions for the general population of illicit users is probably less than 5 percent). LSD is not addictive in the usual sense; it is taken intermittently and usually gradually discontinued. The hallucinogens produce no physical dependence but pose hazards in individuals, and flashbacks of effects may occur even months after the last dose (attributed by some physicians to hysterical reactions associated with unresolved conflicts). The lethal dose is so high that no human deaths have been reported from overdosage.

MODULE VII: 1

Exercise: Expectancy (VIE) Theory Applied to a Personal Decision

Objectives:

1.   To demonstrate VIE theory with personal decision situations.

2.   To increase awareness of the factors involved in motivating workers.

Instructor's Role: To monitor dyad experience, explain VIE theory, and lead large group discussion.

Operating Procedures, Hints, and Cautions:

1.   When explaining the theory, try to think of examples that might apply to this particular group. Tune in to the issues with which people in the group might be dealing.

2.   Encourage participants to take the exercises seriously and to pick a partner with whom they feel comfortable.

3.   Don't listen to the dyads closely. This will only inhibit the participants.

Alternatives and Variations:

If you do not wish to take the time for dyad exchanges, you can go through an example with the whole class before explaining VIE theory. You might ask the class of nurses how they picked their nursing program. You can outline outcomes and expectancies. Finally, you can discuss the limitations of the theory after constructing the expectancy table. Participants will usually agree that they didn't go through this process when deciding.

Concluding Points:

1.   VIE theory rests on assumptions similar to rational economic theory: that people search for alternatives, consciously select outcomes, and weigh each alternative in relation to each outcome and assess probabilities.

2.   Current research shows moderate support for VIE theory as a motivational theory.

<u>Reading for Preparation</u>:

Lawler III, E.E. (1973) <u>Motivation in Work Organizations</u>. Monterey, CA:
    Brooks/Cole.
Lawler III, E.E., Nadler, D.A., and Cammann, C. (1979) <u>Organizational
    Assessment: Perspectives on the Measurement of Organizational Behavior
    and the Quality of Working Life</u>. New York: Wiley-Interscience.
Vroom, V. (1964) <u>Work and Motivation</u>. New York: Wiley
Wanous, J.P. (1977) Organizational entry: Newcomers moving from outside to
    inside. <u>Psychological Bulletin</u>, 84:601.

MODULE VII: 2

Exercise: Goal Setting With Employees: Application to a Problem

Objectives:

1. To improve skills in setting goals with employees.

2. To teach a management by objectives approach to problem solving.

Instructor's Role: To monitor dyad interactions, facilitate large group discussion and clarify the goal setting process.

Operating Procedures, Hints, and Cautions:

1. Have a clear understanding of the management by objectives approach to motivation and problem solving.

2. Encourage participants to select problems that are important to them, but not too personal to discuss in class.

3. Be sure that participants avoid the pitfalls in goal setting.

Alternatives and Variations:

1. You may want to provide a suitable example for the class before dividing into dyads.

2. Participants can discuss the questions in small groups rather than the larger group if there is a large class. This will allow more participation by more class members.

Concluding Points:

1. Management by objectives is a philosophical approach to improving organizational effectiveness. This exercise only touches one small part of that approach.

2. MBO is popular because it (a) is results-oriented, (b) follows a natural cycle of planning and following through to performance evaluation, (c) can be used at any or all levels in the organization, and (d) is fairly straightforward and logical.

Reading for Preparation:

Carrol, S., and Tosi, H. (1980) <u>Management by Objectives</u>, (2nd ed.). New York: MacMillan.

French, W.L., and Hollman, R.W. (1975) Management by objectives: The team approach, <u>California Management Review</u>, 17(3):13.

Jamieson, B. (1973) Behavioral problems with management by objectives. <u>Academy of Management Journal</u>, 16: 496.

Morrissey, G.L. (1972) <u>Appraisal and Development Through Objectives and Results</u>. Reading, MA: Addison-Wesley.

Odiorne, G. (1968) <u>Management Decisions by Objectives</u>. Englewood Cliffs, N.J.: Prentice-Hall

MODULE VII: 3

Exercise: Giving Praise and Feedback

Objectives:
1. To provide practice in giving positive reinforcement to employees.

2. To examine the individual's strengths and weaknesses in praising others.

3. To provide an opportunity for individuals to discuss their strengths within a group.

Instructor's Role: To monitor triad role plays and small group discussion.

Operating Procedures, Hints, and Cautions:

1. Be familiar with positive reinforcement and motivational theories.

2. Read the exercise in the Student Workbook.

3. Some participants may have difficulty or discomfort in talking about themselves positively to others. Remind them that discussing their accomplishments is not bragging, but rather using a good assertive skill.

Alternatives and Variations:

The behavioral rehearsal method is well suited to this exercise. Do only three or four role plays and expect that some participants will have more difficulty talking about themselves positively in a larger group.

Concluding Points:

1. Finding something to praise for some employees may be difficult. However, finding something, even if it is small, is a step toward building a relationship.

2. When praising an employee, always allow time for it "to sink in."

3. Sincerity and genuineness are essential. Discuss how nonverbal behavior is an indicator of sincerity.

Reading for Preparation:

Bolton, R. (1979) People Skills. Englewood Cliffs, NJ: Prentice-Hall.
Reece, B.L. and Brandt, R. (1981) Effective Human Relations in Business.
    Boston: Houghton Mifflin.

MODULE VIII: 1

Exercise: Setting Priorities: An In-Basket Experience

Objectives:

1. To learn how to set priorities on management tasks.

2. To understand the role of time management in successful nurse management.

Instructor's Role: To lead group discussion and provide directions/classification.

Operating Procedures, Hints, and Cautions:

1. Participants usually enjoy the challenge of this task and will have several ways of approaching it. Many will not finish the task in the allotted time, become frustrated, or work from first to last without scanning first. You may have to reemphasize that time management means doing the tasks within deadlines.

2. Be sure to monitor the 30 minute time period carefully.

3. Be familiar with basic concepts of time management.

4. In conducting the discussion, the following points are useful to make:
    a. Participants should scan the entire set of memos before acting. This is the best strategy to prevent a misplaced focus on unimportant items.
    b. Another common mistake is to act on each piece of paper. This is not necessary as it wastes time.
    c. Delegation is important and should be used whenever possible.
    d. Final action to get rid of a memo is generally best. However, some items may be put on hold that will "take care of themselves."
    e. Nurse managers should get in the habit of making up a daily "to do" list using the prioritizing method here for time management.

5. The following is the proper sequence for the memos:
    Memo #1 A   (see the family)
         2   B   (delegate)
         3   C   (refer to staff meeting
         4   A or C (complete in am)
         5   C   (schedule Ann to attend)
         6   C   (schedule staff meeting)
         7   C   (discuss with Kim)
         8   A   (verify date and process)
         9   C
        10   A   (see patient)

11	A	(review schedule and call employee)
12	A	(schedule meeting with Bev or talk to Bev)
13	A	(schedule meeting with dietary)
14	A	
15	B	(delegate to Ann) or C

Alternatives and Variations:

You may want to assign the background information and the in-basket as advance preparation for class. Although you can't monitor the time limit, you will have more time in class for discussion.

Concluding Points:

1. Other time management techniques include delegating, postponing, and discarding. These can be applied to all aspects of life, home, social engagements, and work.

2. The benefits of time management include the following:
   a. Reducing stress
   b. Improving efficiency
   c. Reducing role overload
   d. Getting more accomplished in less time
   e. Getting the important things done
   f. Developing subordinates through delegation
   g. Freeing time for personal development

3. Delegation requires special considerations. The following may be helpful:
   a. Review plans daily and assign what you can to others.
   b. Assign as many tasks as possible, expecting that there will be some mistakes at first.
   c. Let others know to whom you assigned the task.
   d. Give proper authority to go with the responsibility for the task.
   e. Monitor progress with specific completion times and followup meetings.
   f. Delegate by results, not means. Let people develop their own means and determine success by results only.

Reading for Preparation:

Douglas, E. and Goodwin, P.H. (1980) Successful Time Management for Hospital Administrators. New York: Amacom.

Lakeiu, A. (1973) How to Get Control of Your Time and Life. New York: Signet.

Douglas, M.E. (1978) The Time Management Workbook, Time Management Center, St. Louis, MO.

Bliss, E.C. (1976) <u>Getting Things Done, The ABC's of Time Management</u>, New
    York: Scribner.
Oncken, W., Jr. and Wass, D.L. (1974) Management Time: Who's Got the Monkey?
    <u>Harvard Business Review</u>, 5, 105.
Gibson, J.L., Ivancevich, J.W. and Donnelly, J.H., (1988) <u>Organizations:</u>
    <u>Behavior, Structure, Processes</u>, Hazelwood, IL., Richard A. Irwin, Inc.

MODULE VIII: 2

Exercise: How to Handle Time Wasters

Objectives:

1. To teach skills in handling common time wasters for managers (e.g., phone calls and drop-in visitors).

2. To increase awareness of the need for time management.

Instructor's Role: To monitor triad role plays and lead large group discussion.

Operating Procedures, Hints, and Cautions:

1. You may want to demonstrate to the class how to handle phone calls and drop-in visitors. Select a participant and brief him/her before the demonstration. Use realistic situations to which the class members can relate. Allow the class to critique your role play. Encourage constructive feedback and discussion.

2. Think of several ideas for role play to give to participants who request this of you, but encourage them to think of their own ideas first.

3. Some participants may have difficulty being assertive in these situations. This provides an excellent opportunity to discuss assertiveness as a necessary skill for nurse managers. (See Module IV.)

Alternatives and Variations:

To reduce the time needed for this exercise, the instructor can role-play both situations in front of the class and lead the discussion without triad role play. However, participants will not get the benefits of practice.

Concluding Points:

Controlling time wasters is only one part of time management. For managers, other aspects included analyzing your time, setting priorities, organizing your time for better results, developing good time use habits, and influencing others to use their time more efficiently.

Reading for Preparation:

Douglas, M.E. Creative use of time. (1975) The Personnel Administrator.
Goldfein, D. (1977) Every Woman's Guide to Time Management.
    Less Lemmes Publishing.

MODULE VIII: 3

Exercise: Delegation for Results

Objectives:

1.   To understand the roles of manager and subordinate in the delegation process.

2.   To identify successful methods and stumbling blocks for delegation.

Instructor's Role: To direct small group experience, helping leaders and observers when needed.

Operating Procedures, Hints, and Cautions:

1.   Construct from cardboard one puzzle (pictured below) for each group in your class.

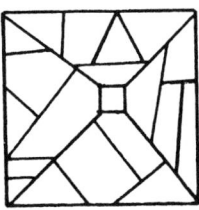

2.   Make sure operators read only their instructions. Pay special attention to observers--make sure they know their role.

3.   Pay attention to the time for each activity especially the five minute operator briefing by managers.

4.   Encourage participants to "get into" their roles.

5.   Be certain the participants understand the rules of the exercise. Do not allow any communication about the square between operators during assembly.

Alternatives and Variations:

1.   The time for the task can be varied by making the hollow square simpler or more complex. However, if you simplify, there will be less time for the observers to rate quality of assembly.

Concluding Points:

1.   Discuss the importance of delegation in nursing management.

2.   Discuss authority vs. responsibility in delegation.

3.   Connect delegation to time management.

Reading for Preparation:

Bliss, E. (1976) <u>Getting Things Done: The ABS's of Time Management</u>, N.Y.,
      Scriber's.
McCoukey, D. (1974) <u>No-Nonsense Delegation</u>, N.Y. AMACOM.
Wineben, S. (1983) <u>The Organized Executive</u>, W.W. Norton & Co., N.Y.

MODULE VIII: 4

Exercise: Assessing Stress Levels and Reducing Stress

Objectives:

    1.   To encourage identification of stressors.
    2.   To increase awareness of coping strategies.
    3.   To help establish goals for stress reduction.
    4.   To stimulate thinking about managerial stress.

Instructor's Role: To provide guidance in self-assessment of stress levels and to create an individualized stress reduction plan.

Operating Procedures, Hints and Cautions:

    1.   Be familiar with the literature on stress, managerial stress, and stress reduction methods.

    2.   Read Exercise VIII:4 in the Student Workbook and familiarize yourself with the Stress Tests and Stress Reduction Plan.

    3.   Complete the Stress Reduction Plan for yourself in order to better help the participants.

    4.   The scoring procedures for the Stress Tests are as follows:

        a.   Stress Test I is the Life Event Scale by Holmes and Rahe (1967). It is based on the research which shows that life events require physical and emotional adaptation and cause stress. An account of the number and kind of these events in the past 12 months is a remarkable predictor of physical and mental illness.
                Below 150 total points = low risk
                Between 150 and 300 total points = moderate risk
                Over 300 total points = high risk

        b.   Stress Test II is a test of the degree of overload one is experiencing.
                26-40 points = high level
                20-25 points = moderate stress level
                10-19 points = low stress level

        c.   Stress Test III is a test of Type A/B behavior patterns. Items 1, 2, and 3 deal with time urgency. Items 4, 5, and 6 deal with aggressiveness. Items 7 and 8 deal with the tendency to rush into things without properly defined goals. Items 9 and 10 deal with polyphasic behavior (doing several things at once).

                27-40 points = Type A behavior
                20-25 points = moderate Type A behavior

                    20- 0 points = not Type A

    d.   Stress Test IV is a test of the anxious reactivity of
           behavior. It means the degree of hypersensitivity of a
           person in stress situations.
                26-40 points = high anxious reactivity
                20-25 points = average
                20-0 points = low anxious reactivity

5.   Be prepared to help participants interpret their scores and
       complete their stress reduction plans.

6.   Remember that the exercise requires considerable introspection and
       creativity in looking at alternatives. Participants may get
       "stuck" or frustrated and will need support.

7.   Participants will be sharing personal information. You may want
       to address this issue in the beginning to help them feel more
       comfortable.

Alternatives and Variations

Sharing information about the stress reduction plan can be done in
dyads. This will reduce the time needed for the exercise and may reduce
participants' fears of self-disclosure. However, the evaluation may be less
valuable and alternatives may be missed.

Concluding Points:

1.   An 80% chance of serious illness is present among those who score
       over 300 on the Holmes and Rahe Scale.

2.   In 1900, women lived an average of two years longer than men. In
       1970, the difference was 7.7 years. By 2000, the gap is estimated
       to be more than 12 years.

3.   Individuals who live balanced lives with physical, spiritual,
       social, intellectual and personal activities cope more effectively
       with stress.

4.   Regular physical exercise is one of the best preventions of stress
       related mental/physical disorders.

5.   Self-awareness, i.e., knowing your cognitive and interpersonal
       styles and your limits, is highly correlated with successful
       coping with stress.

6.   Managers primarily face time, situational, and interpersonal
       stresses.

Reading for Preparation:

Selye, H. (1976) <u>The Stress of Life</u> (2nd Ed.) New York: McGraw-Hill.
Kobosa, S.C. (1970) Stressful life events, personality and health: An inquiry into hardiness. <u>Journal of Personality and Social Psychology</u>, 37:1.
Cooper, C.L. and Davidson, M.J. (1982) The high cost of stress on women managers. <u>Organizational Dynamics</u>, 11:44.
Girdano, D. and Everly, G. (1979) <u>Controlling Stress and Tension: A Holistic Approach</u>. Englewood Cliffs: Prentice-Hall.

MODULE IX: 1

Exercise: Developing a Structured Interview Guide.

Objectives:

1. To increase awareness of the types of information that can be obtained in the selection interview.

2. To provide practice in constructing a structured interview guide.

3. To help participants identify some of the advantages of structured interviews.

Instructor's Role: To monitor small group experience and lead large group discussion.

Operating Procedures, Hints, and Cautions:

1. Be familiar with the exercise procedure and the different forms used in developing the structured interview guide in the Student Workbook.

2. Be thoroughly familiar with the Job Description for Nurse Manager.

3. When participants are outlining the job requirements, encourage them to think in terms of mental ability, skill, job knowledge and traits. Be careful of traits and help participants to define them behaviorally. It helps if participants write the headings "task," "skill/ability," and "question" across the top of a page.

4. Explain Realistic Job Preview (RJP) to the participants if they do not have prior knowledge. Giving job information to the applicant is important. Research has shown that giving realistic job preview information to applicants will result in increased job satisfaction and lower turnover. However, this should be done at the end of the interview so that the information will not guide the applicant's answers during the interview. Generally, realistic job previews are institution- or job-specific. However, for this exercise, instruct the participants to derive the realistic job preview information for the structured guide from experience of group members on similar jobs. An example is provided in Module IX: 1 of the Student Workbook.

Alternatives and Variations:

1. To reduce the time in class needed for the exercise, instruct students to complete steps 2 and 3 in the Student Workbook and bring their responses to class.

2. Understanding of the Realistic Job Preview can be enhanced by using the example that is included in the Student Workbook (Module

IX: 1). This will work best if most participants have been or are employed.

Concluding Points:

A good interview requires an adequate job analysis. Point out other requirements for a good interview, such as those suggested in Model IX: 2 of the Student Workbook. Discuss the validity of the interview. Why is it dubious at best?

Reading for Preparation:

Arvey, R.D. (1979) Fairness in Selecting Employees. Reading, MA: Addison-Wesley.
Heneman, H.G., et al (1975) Interviewer validity as a function of interview structure, biographical data and interviewee order. Journal of Applied Psychology, 60:748.
Arvey, R.D. and Campion, J.E. (1982) The employment interview: A summary and review of recent research. Personnel Psychology, 35:281
Goodale, J.G. (1982) The Fine Art of Interviewing, Englewood Cliffs, N.J.: Prentice-Hall

MODULE IX: 2

Exercise: Conducting an Interview

Objectives:

1. To provide the opportunity to practice skills in interviewing an applicant for a nursing management position.

2. To generate feedback for participants on how they are seen by others as an applicant in an interview.

3. To increase awareness of one's strengths and weaknesses as an interviewer.

Instructor's Role: To monitor the triad role plays and lead large group discussion.

Operating Procedures, Hints, and Cautions:

1. Be sure that participants bring their interview guides to class. Each person should have a copy of his/her group's completed interview guide. If Exercise IX-1 was not done, you may want to develop and provide a completed interview guide.

2. No groups should have more than four members as this will lengthen the task; however, if there is a group with four members, instruct them to interview for 15 minutes only.

3. Be familiar with the forms provided in the Student Workbook.

4. Remind participants that they only have a limited time to interview in class. To avoid a "surface" interview, tell participants to decide in advance to probe in one or two areas only. This will give them experience in data gathering. Otherwise, there is a tendency for participants to skip lightly over all topics.

5. Be thoroughly familiar with the issues related to use of the interview as a selection device.

6. Remember that participants are likely to feel anxious, as if the role play were a real interview. This will happen if the instructor encourages the interviewer to set up the situation as real as possible.

Alternatives and Variations:

1. If students have not completed Module IX: Exercise 1, instruct them to read it and prepare an Interview Guide, using the Job Description for Nurse Manager (located in Student Workbook, Module IX: 1) prior to class. Expect participants to have questions

about their interview guides, which should be addressed before beginning the role plays.

2.   It is not recommended that participants work in pairs to reduce the time needed for the exercise. This prevents them from getting adequate feedback.

Concluding Points:

Discuss the Tips for Applicants in detail. Many participants will find these relevant to their personal situations. Balance the discussion in the direction of the interviewer, since most participants will be required to interview applicants in their future jobs as well.

Reading for Preparation:

Arvey, R.D. (1979) Fairness in Selecting Employees. Reading, MA: Addison-Wesley.

Arvey, R.D. and Campion, J.E. (1982) The employment interview: A summary and review of recent research. Personnel Psychology, 35:281.

Goodale, J.G. (1982) The Fine Art of Interviewing. Englewood Cliffs, NJ: Prentice-Hall.

Heneman, H.G., et al (1975) Interviewer validity as a function of interview structure, biographical data, and interviewee order. Journal of Applied Psychology, 60:748.

Stewart, C.J. and Cash, W.B. (1985), Interviewing: Principles and Practice, Dubuque, IA: William C. Brown Co.

MODULE X: 1

Exercise: On-the-Job Training (OJT)

Objectives:

1. To build skills in teaching others using an on-the-job training technique.

2. To provide the opportunity to explore the strengths/weaknesses of OJT.

3. To provide practice in development of key behaviors for OJT.

Instructor's Role: To direct the dyad exercise, facilitate discussion, and monitor development of key behaviors.

Operating Procedures, Hints, and Cautions

1. Do not tell participants that they will be doing this exercise because they should not read it. Just tell them to bring their Student Workbook to class on the day of this exercise.

2. Be thoroughly familiar with the Student Workbook instructions for this exercise in order to guide the participants.

3. Bring 5-8 sheets of 8 x 11 paper for each participant.

4. Learn how to make the paper cup presented in Module X: 1 of the Student Workbook.

5. Be familiar with concepts. Note Figures X:1-A, X:1-B, and X:1-C are provided to assist in any discussion of social learning theory, behavior modeling and principles of learning you wish to provide.

6. Do not help the participants to fold the paper cup unless it begins to take longer than the allotted time. Then, suggest you will show them how to do it if they all agree that learning something from written instructions (i.e., technical manual) is very difficult.

7. Remind the trainers to use their key behaviors for OJT.

8. When all trainees have learned the manual task, ask the "trainers" to have the "trainees" fold one or two more cups. Discuss the concept of overlearning.

9. Ask the trainers by which method they would have preferred to learn this task (hopefully they will say OJT). Have the trainers show the trainees how they learned the task.

10. In the social skills training, explain the process of step 9 in

the _Student Workbook_ (Module X:1) to the participants.

11. When all the trainees have learned the three steps of giving recognition, explain the importance of generalization in teaching social skills, i.e., social skills are generalized by practicing the skills with different people and in various contexts. (Practice giving recognition for a different performance to a different person.)

12. When teaching participants to develop key behaviors for a specific task in OJT, help them to select a workable task. Be familiar with the Job Breakdown Sheet (Module X:1 in the _Student Workbook_) and the process of generating key behaviors for OJT.

13. In the discussion, refer to Figure X-1C concerning attitude change and behavior change.

Alternatives and Variations

1. In teaching the social skills, an option is to have each trainer select two trainees and teach one trainee to give recognition to the second trainee. Using the On-the-Job Training Key Behaviors, the trainer does the three steps of giving recognition to the second trainee in Key Behaviors 2 and 4. During Key Behaviors 5, 6, and 7, the first trainee does the three steps of giving recognition to the second trainee. Then the two trainees switch roles and the trainer teaches again.

2. To reduce the time needed for the exercise, the development of key behaviors (steps 13, 14, and 15 in the _Student Workbook_) can be eliminated. However, the instructor should include discussion of the Job Breakdown Sheet located in Module X:1 of the _Student Workbook_.

Concluding Points:

This is a critical exercise which should always be used to teach nurses how to teach others.

Reading for Preparation

Bandura, A. (1977) _Social Learning Theory_. Englewood Cliffs, NJ: Prentice-Hall.

Decker, P.J. (1980) Effects of symbolic coding and rehearsal in behavior modeling training. _Journal of Applied Psychology_, 65:627.

Craig, R.L. (ed.) (1976) _Training and Development Handbook_, (2nd ed). New York: McGraw-Hill, Chapter 32.

Manz, C.C. and Sims, H.P., Jr. (1981) Vicarious learning: The influence on modeling on organizational behavior. _Academy of Management Review_, 6:105.

Decker, P.J. and Nathan, B. (1985) _Behavior Modeling Training: Principles and Applications_. New York: Praeger.

Wexley, K. and Latham, G.P. (1981) _Developing and Training Human Resources in Organizations_. Glenview, IL: Scott, Foresman.

MODULE X: 2

Exercise: Day-to-Day Coaching of Employees

Objectives:

1.   To build skill in day-to-day coaching of employees.

2.   To build skills in diagnosing employee performance problems.

Instructor's Role: To lead discussion, monitor role plays, and demonstrate a coaching session.

Operating Procedures, Hints and Cautions

1.   Be prepared to show the class how to coach an employee. Brief a participant before class and/or go through the role play several times. Don't try to make it perfect, however, you should follow the key behaviors as much as possible. Allow participants to be critical and to offer suggestions. This will help them in the trial role plays. For the demonstration, select an example from your experience with an employee with a performance deficiency.

2.   Encourage participants to play the roles using the suggestions given in the introduction of this book. The employee should be "real" and not compliant.

3.   Be sure to include discussion time for diagnosing performance problems.

Alternatives and Variations:

1.   You can omit the demonstration if you think that participants can work easily in triads. This will save time but also reduce the opportunity for participants to develop critical skills.

2.   If you have access to a videotape recorder, you may want to videotape a coaching session to use for class demonstration.

3.   Participants who have worked as nurse managers may want to come up with their own performance deficiency problems with staff.

Concluding Points:

Knowledge of expectancy (VIE) theory is assumed for this exercise. Therefore, a brief overview of VIE theory may be helpful.

Reading for Preparation:

Campbell, J.P. and Pritchard, R.D. (1976) Motivation theory in industrial and organizational psychology. In M. Dunnette (ed.), Handbook of Industrial and Organizational Psychology. Chicago: Rand McNally.

Fischer, C.D. (1979) Transmission of positive and negative feedback to subordinates: A laboratory investigation. Journal of Applied Psychology, 15:533.

Goodale, J.G. (1982) The Fine Art of Interviewing. (Chapters 4 & 6). Englewood Cliffs, NJ: Prentice Hall.

Larson, J.R. (1981) Some hypotheses about the causes of supervisory performance feedback behavior. Proceedings of the 41st Annual Academy of Management Meeting, San Diego.

Lawler, E.E. (1973) Motivation in Work Organizations. Monterey, CA: Brooks Cole.

Mitchell, T.R. (1974) Expectancy models of job satisfaction, occupational preference, and effort: A theoretical, methodological, and empirical approach. Psychological Bulletin, 81:1053.

Nadler, D.A. (1979) The effects of feedback on task group behavior: A review of the experimental research. Organizational Behavior and Human Performance, 23:309.

MODULE XI: 1

Exercise: Handling a Discipline Problem

Objectives:

1.   To provide the opportunity to practice handling a discipline problem.

2.   To increase awareness of the complexity and process of disciplining employees.

3.   To provide feedback on performance in a discipline situation.

Instructor's Role: To monitor triad role plays and lead large group discussion.

Operating Procedures, Hints, and Cautions:

1.   Be familiar with the issues and problems in the use of discipline in an organization.

2.   Encourage a discussion of using authority and delivering negative information to employees. This is a common problem area for new managers, i.e., a reluctance to exert authority when needed, which results in resentment, decreased motivation, or lack of respect from subordinates. The right balance of firmness with caring is difficult to attain in discipline. Feedback from others is especially helpful in identifying strengths and weaknesses in communicating assertively but with concern and a positive approach.

Alternatives and Variations

1.   This exercise is well suited to the behavioral rehearsal method. If the group is small, i.e., a maximum of 15 members, behavioral rehearsal gives the instructor the advantage of more careful monitoring of the role plays. If behavioral rehearsal is used, have only four or five participants actually role-play in one class period.

2.   If participants want to derive their own situations for role play, encourage them to do so. This will enhance involvement.

Concluding Points:

Many participants will express some difficulty in discipline. Help them to sort out the major issues of proper timing, appropriateness of discipline, emotional reactions, use of power, etc. Encourage participants to evaluate both verbal and nonverbal communication in the role plays. For example, a participant may verbally state the appropriate words but use a weak or shaky voice that detracts from the message.

<u>Reading for Preparation</u>:

Beletz, E.E., (1986) Discipline: Establishing just cause for correction,
    <u>Nursing Management</u>, 17:63-67.
Blanchard, K. and Johnson, S. (1984) <u>The One Minute Manager</u>. New York:
    Berkley Books.

MODULE XI: 2

Exercise: Writing Critical Incidents/Noteworthy Behaviors

Objectives:

1. To teach skills in writing noteworthy behaviors effectively.

2. To increase understanding of the role of the critical incident technique (CIT) in performance appraisal.

Instructor's Role: To lead large group discussion, enact a role play, and monitor small group experience.

Operating Procedures, Hints, and Cautions:

1. Be prepared to explain the reasons for the answers to the CIT quiz. Include an explanation of the difference between behavior and attitude. The following are the answers with explanations.

   1. No. "Sloppily" is not defined.
   2. No. "Very honest" is not specific.
   3. No. An explanation of her actions is required.
   4. No. The word "weak" is too vague.
   5. Yes.
   6. No. This is an interpretation, not description.
   7. Yes.
   8. No. "Poor attitude" is not explained.
   9. Yes.
   10. No. "Rarely" does not tell how often.
   11. Yes
   12. No. "Pleasant" is too vague.
   13. No. "Behaviors are not named.
   14. No. "upset" is not explained.
   15. No. "Too much" is not specific.
   16. Yes.
   17. No. Behavior is not reported.
   18. Yes. States what _he_ did although his statement is not adequate description of her behavior.
   19. No. Interpretation not observation.
   20. Yes.

2. Monitor the small groups carefully and provide assistance when needed. Sometimes participants will see and hear different things. To avoid an argument, have your role-play script written out prior to class. Pick a participant to play the other role and coach this person to follow the script. This can be done briefly prior to the class meeting.

3. Be prepared to discuss behavioral observation scales versus trait based scales.

Alternatives and Variations:

1.   If the class is small, remain as a whole group when discussing the
      written critical incidents.

2.   Try enacting two shorter incidents, one positive and one negative.

Concluding Points:

1.   Keeping critical incidents provides good feedback in a performance
      review session.

2.   All behaviorally based rating forms (e.g., BOS) that are developed
      from critical incidents have been shown to be reliable as measured
      by inter-observer, test-retest and internal consistency methods.

Reading for Preparation:

Latham, G.P. and Wexley, K.N. (1981). Increasing Productivity
      Through Performance Appraisal. Reading, MA: Addison-Wesley.

MODULE XI: 3

Exercise: Conducting a Performance Appraisal Interview

Objectives:

1.   To provide experience in conducting a performance appraisal interview.

2.   To increase awareness of types of performance appraisal instruments and interviews.

Instructor's Role: To monitor triad role plays and lead large group discussion.

Operating Procedures, Hints, and Cautions:

1.   Be familiar with the types of performance appraisal instruments and the most effective methods for performance review.

2.   Be prepared to encourage participants to complete the performance appraisal evaluation. Try not to be judgmental or to make their decision; rather, guide the participant toward his/her own conclusions.

3.   Visit the group of participants who play Susan Allen while they review their parts in another room. Help them to take on her "personality" for the interview.

4.   The discussion time should include information on performance appraisal instruments provided by the instructor. Encourage a critical examination of the usefulness of the instrument used here.

Alternatives and Variations:

1.   The performance review can be done by two participants while the rest of the group observes. You can add to the role play by being the "alter ego" for either of the participants, by adding what you think the person is feeling but not saying. This allows for more input from others but should not be done if the group is larger than 15 members.

2.   Participants can discuss the questions in small groups of six or nine members rather than in the whole group. This may save time.

Concluding Points:

1.   Behavior-oriented performance appraisal instruments provide better feedback to the employee.

2.   Listening and understanding are your best recourse when the employee becomes defensive during an interview.

3. Focusing on job performance, not personality factors, is a must if you want to minimize defensiveness.

4. Salary reviews should be kept separate from developmental review if possible.

5. Feelings play a big role in performance reviews.

6. Critical incidents can be a great support during a review and should be kept on positives and negatives.

Reading for Preparation:

Clark, M.D. (1982) Performance Appraisal, Nursing Management, 13:27-29.
    Goodale, J.G. (1982) The Fine Art of Interviewing. Englewood Cliffs, NJ: Prentice-Hall.
Latham, G.P. and Wexley, K.N. (1982) Increasing Productivity Through Performance Appraisal. Reading, MA: Addison-Wesley.

MODULE XII: 1

Exercise: Handling and Preventing Grievances

Objectives:

1. To provide practice in handling an employee grievance.

2. To increase awareness of ways to prevent grievances.

3. To provide a framework for handling grievances.

Instructor's Role: To monitor role plays and small group discussion.

Operating Procedures, Hints, and Cautions:

1. Be familiar with research on employee grievances in union and nonunion situations.

2. Encourage the participants to "get into" their roles fully.

3. Be sure participants fully understand the key behaviors.

Alternatives and Variations:

The instructor may first role-play handling a grievance with a participant before the whole group. This will serve as a model. The whole class can be the observers and the instructor leads the feedback discussion. This can be in addition to triad role plays or a substitution. However, if the triads are eliminated, the practice part of the exercise is diminished.

Concluding Points:

Over 95% of all collective bargaining agreements contain a grievance procedure that ends in a binding arbitration. You may want to share the example of a typical union grievance procedure with the class (Example XII-A). This will encourage a comparison between nonunion and union grievance handling.

Example XII-A

Grievance Procedure

Step 1. The aggrieved employee and shop steward shall meet and discuss the grievance with the employee's immediate supervisor. If not satisfactorily resolved in three (3) working days, the grievance shall be placed in writing and Step 2 should be taken.

The above step does not prohibit or preclude filing of a grievance by the grievance committee if the union considers it necessary. In such cases, the grievance committee shall specify the employee or employees alleged to have been aggrieved.

Step 2. The shop steward shall meet with the department head for discussion of the grievance. If not satisfactorily adjusted in three (3) working days, Step 3 should be taken.

Step 3. The grievance committee consisting of (4) members appointed by the union shall discuss the grievance with the administrator or his/her appointed representative. A representative of the national union may be present at this meeting. The aggrieved employee may also be present.

Step 4. If the company and the union cannot agree on a settlement of any grievance or dispute within 72 hours after Step 3 has been taken, the dispute between the parties may be submitted to arbitration as set forth in paragraph (b) below, provided that either party has given written notice requesting arbitration within 15 days following completion of the final meeting held under Step 3. In this event, the arbitration procedure set forth below shall prevail.

The parties shall designate a mutually satisfactory arbitrator. In the event they fail to agree upon such arbitrator within three (3) days after arbitration is requested as aforesaid, the Federal Mediation and Conciliation Service shall, at the request of either party, furnish the institution and the union with a list for the selection of an arbitrator. The list furnished by the FMCS, however, shall be restricted to the geographic area of New Jersey and metropolitan New York. The arbitrator shall hear the matter in dispute as soon as possible and render an award thereon in writing. The award of the arbitrator shall be final and conclusively binding on the parties.

An attempt to settle all disputes and grievances by consultations in the manner hereinabove outlined shall be a condition precedent to arbitration and shall be of the essence of this Agreement. A demand that a matter be submitted to arbitration must in all cases take place within 35 working days after the occurrence giving rise to the dispute or grievance in question. All costs of arbitration shall be borne equally by the company and the union, except that each party shall procure the attendance of witnesses at its own cost and expense.

Grievance within the meaning of the grievance procedure and this arbitration clause shall consist only of disputes about the interpretation or application of particular clauses of the Agreement and about alleged violations of the Agreement. The arbitrator shall have no power to add to, subtract from, or modify wage schedules or modify any of the terms of this Agreement, nor shall the arbitrator substitute discretion for that of the company or the union, nor exercise any responsibility or function of the company or union.

The company agrees to pay those employees involved in the above grievance procedure for all time lost from their regularly scheduled shift.

Reading for Preparation:

Bean, J.J. & Laliberty, R. (1977) Understanding Hospital Labor Relations. Reading, MA: Addison-Wesley.

Beletz, E.E., (1977) Some Pointers for Grievance Handlers, Supervisor Nurse,8:12-14.

Trotta, M.S. (1976) Handling Grievances: A Guide for Management and Labor. Washington, DC: Bureau of National Affairs, Inc.

MODULE XII: 2

Exercise: Issues in Labor Relations

Objectives:

    1.   To facilitate analysis and understanding of key issues in nursing labor relations.

    2.   To provide practice in decision making in labor issues.

Instructor's Role: To facilitate group discussion of cases.

Operating Procedures, Hints, and Cautions:

    1.   Do not assign more than two cases per class period.

    2.   Familiarize yourself with the Wagner Act.

    3.   Read each case and discussion question before class. Formulate your own answers. Check the law!

    4.   Case discussion question responses are at the end of these instructions.

Alternatives and Variations:

    Do not skip the individual written analysis. It may be graded but need not be. This represents the students' practice: the class discussion is feedback. If you shortcut the written analysis, you shortchange the student's learning process.

    The discussion may occur in groups of 5 to 10, but would be better with the whole class participating and you facilitating discussion.

Concluding Points:

    1.   Do not be quick to solve the problem--let the students discuss it and defend what they have written.

Reading for Preparation:

Dilts, D.A. and Deitsch, C.R. (1983) Labor Relations. New York: MacMillian.
Fossum, J.A. (1982) Labor Relations Dallas, TX: Business Publications.
Schoen, S.H. and Hilgert, R.L. (1982) Cases in Collective Bargaining and Industrial Relations. (4th ed). Homewood, IL: Irwin.

CASE 1

MCGRATH HOSPITAL

The McGrath Hospital case will offer students a good example of how a personnel director or any manager <u>should</u> <u>not</u> deal with a union organizing campaign. Pete Watson, apparently unfamiliar and unaccustomed to any type of union efforts in his hospital, is reacting rather than having a sound strategy for meeting the union's organization attempt.

Union organizers have a legal right to distribute literature outside of the premises of a company or hospital they are trying to organize. The fact that a number of employees at McGrath Hospital are complaining to management about being "bothered" by union organizers should be approached by management cautiously and sensitively. However, Personnel Director Pete Watson reacts with a very strongly worded letter that could backfire on him by mobilizing sentiments of employees to be sympathetic to union organizers. In his letter, Watson tells employees to contact their supervisors for answers to questions. There is no evidence in the case that the supervisors would know how to respond to any questions the employees may have.

The union committee members are angry, perhaps justifiably so. The long-service employees think that Watson's letter was quite unfair in labeling them as "strangers." At the end of the case, the union organizing committee and their local union president, Mr. Brown, are to discuss the situation with Mr. Watson. However, Mr. Watson is reluctant to meet with Mr. Brown as part of the committee meeting. Here, too, Mr. Watson is on dangerous grounds, politically as well as legally. It appears that Mr. Watson is again reacting rather than thinking calmly about how he can meet the union challenge positively.

CASE 2

THE HOSPITAL'S WITHDRAWAL OF RECOGNITION
AND REFUSAL TO BARGAIN WITH A NURSES UNION

(Windham Community Memorial Hospital and Registered Nurses Unit 62 (Connecticut Nurses Association)

The Administrative Law Judge, the National Labor Relations Board, and the Court of Appeals (Second Circuit-New York) all held in favor of the union. Specifically, the hospital had violated Sections 8 (a) (5) and 8 (a) (1) of the Labor Management Relations Act when, during negotiations for a new collective bargaining contract, it refused to bargain with and withdrew recognition from a union representing its registered nurses, despite the hospital's contention that its refusal to bargain was a proper response to the union's alleged preconditional offer to return to the bargaining table and that its withdrawal of recognition was based on serious good faith doubt of the union's majority status. Concerning the refusal to bargain, the Court commented:

The Hospital did not meet with the Union to voice its objections to the imposition of the alleged conditions, nor did it inform the Union that it would not negotiate under those conditions. Instead of merely refusing to bargain until the alleged conditions were withdrawn, the Hospital chose immediately to withdraw recognition from the Union. Even under the Hospital's version of the August 23rd conversation, this was not an appropriate response. Then, unless the withdrawal of recognition was justifiable under some other theory, it clearly constituted a "refusal to bargain" within the meaning of Section 8 (a) (5) of the Act.

Concerning the majority status of the union, the Administrative Law Judge, the National Labor Relations Board and the Court of Appeals all held that the hospital had not shown affirmatively that the union did not have a majority status on August 23, 1976. The Court commented:

Instead of providing proof, the Hospital merely formulates a presumption of its own: that no replacement employee supports the Union. This presumption is equally, if not more, assailable than the NLRB's; many workers might well be pro-Union but might need the job or might reject the use of strikes in nursing. Considering the propriety of Administrative Law Judge's findings of fact on the question of unit membership and the Hospital's failure to offer objective proof, it is clear that the Hospital did not, by actual proof of lack of majority, rebut the presumption of continued representation status.

The primary ground cited by the Hospital was alleged diminished support for the Union evidenced by the facts that some employees never went out on strike, some strikers returned to work prior to August 23, 1976, and striker replacements had been hired and had been willing to cross the picket line. We find this argument unconvincing. It cannot be presumed that repudiation of a strike or the willingness to cross a picket line is also repudiation of the Union as a bargaining agent. This is especially true in employment which is so closely involved with health and safety; many nurses consider strikes completely improper.

As to remedies, the Administrative Law Judge, the National Labor Relations Board and Court of Appeals all held that the hospital must recognize and bargain with the union and reinstate and/or make whole (in terms of lost pay and benefits) all strikers from August 23, 1976, to their date of their reinstatement (less any income from alternative employment during the applicable period). The Court stated as follows:

It is well-established that an economic strike is converted into an unfair labor practice strike if it is prolonged or aggravated by the employer's unfair labor practice. Reinstatement of all striking employees, with or without back pay, is an appropriate remedy when an unfair labor practice strike is found.

* * *

There is ample evidence to support a finding that the strike was prolonged by the Hospital's action. Withdrawal of recognition from the Union precluded the possibility that the strike could be ended by negotiation. Thus, the concededly economic strike was converted to an unfair labor practice

strike and reinstatement and back pay are entirely appropriate remedies.
(230 NLRB No. 156 -- 99 LRRM 2242-2248)

CASE 62

WHICH DUTY CALLS

(Monroe County Hospital and Civil Service Employees
Association, Monroe Chapter, Local 828)

Decision of the Arbitrator (Irving R. Markowitz):

The parties had submitted the following issue to arbitration:

Was the discharge of Mary Moody for just and sufficient
cause? If not, what shall the remedy be?

The arbitrator held that the discharge of Moody was not for just and
sufficient reason. The hospital was to offer her the position she held prior
to her discharge within 10 working days of this award (March 7, 1979). She
was awarded no back pay from the date of her discharge to the date of her
return to work in accordance with the award. She was considered to be
suspended for that period because of excessive absenteeism. The arbitrator
stated, "If she accepts the award and returns to work within five days after
receiving the hospital's offer, she shall not forfeit her seniority and other
rights under the contract."

The arbitrator stated that a poor attendance record, especially where
the employer is a hospital that requires adequate staffing at all times, is
sufficient reason to terminate an employee. Further, no matter how valid an
employee's excuses may be, no employer should be expected to retain a person
who has been absent at least 10% of her assigned hours.

However, the arbitrator notes, "It is important in cases such as these
that society -- and all those affected -- recognize the individual problems of
an employee." He took cognizance of the "overwhelming problems" with which
Moody was attempting to cope. Moody's daughter was receiving psychological
counseling as was Moody herself, she failed to show "immediate, marked, and
continuous improvement, she will undoubtedly submit herself to permanent
termination." (72LA541)

MODULE XIII: 1

Exercise: Budgeting

Objectives:

1. To develop skill in adjusting salary levels.

2. To practice allocating merit increases based on staff performance.

3. To become aware of the many alternatives in providing salary adjustments.

Instructor's Role: To read scenario with participants and lead discussion of completed reports.

Operating Procedures, Hints, and Cautions:

1. The instructor should complete the Salary Adjustment Report prior to class.

2. The instructor should read the scenario while participants follow along.

3. The participants should be reminded to bring a hand-held calculator to class.

4. The participants should complete the Salary Adjustment Report individually, divide into dyads to compare their answers, and then return to the large group for discussion.

Alternatives and Variations:

Participants may complete the Salary Adjustment Report prior to class. The class can be divided into small groups for discussion of answers and then return to the large group to report on discussion. The instructor can collect the Reports, comment, and then return them to students.

Concluding Points:

1. There are no "right" answers as long as the percentages and totals fall within the guidelines.

2. Salary adjustment is only a part of budgeting but it is significant in contribution to job satisfaction and morale. Also, it is an example of the computations necessary for other aspects of the budget.

Reading for Preparation

Dias, K., Dziekan, N.C. and Willis, B. (1986) Work designs: extended shifts balance workloads and budgets, too! Nursing Management 17:36.

Hittmann, B. (1984) Selling your budget. RN, 47:25.

Knight-Sheen, J.P. (1983) The Medrec Calculator: A New Way to Plan for Nurse Staffing. San Antonio, TX: Medrec Publishing.

Rotkovitch, R. (1981) The nursing director's role in money management. Journal of Nursing Administration, XI, (11-12), 13.

Stevens, B.J. (1975) The Nurse as Executive. Wakefield, MA: Contemporary Publishing.

Stevens, B.J. (1981) What is the executive's role in budgeting for her department? Journal of Nursing Administration, 11:22.

MODULE XIII: 2

Exercise: Staff Scheduling

Objectives:

1. To develop skill in arranging staff schedule.

2. To become aware of the conflicts inherent in scheduling staff time.

3. To increase organizational and planning skills.

Instructor's Role: To read directions to class and explain the key.

Operating Procedures, Hints, and Cautions:

1. The instructor should read the directions aloud while participants follow along reading their own copies.

2. Bring schedule sheet, red pencil, and eraser for each student to class.

3. Exercise is to be completed individually and then discussed in the large group.

4. Go over the form and the participant's decisions thoroughly in class. Be sure every student understands the reasons for each decision.

5. Become very familiar with the Rationale for Answer Key (Figure XIII: 2-A) in order to substantiate the decisions on the Schedule Answer Key (Figure XIII: 2-C).

6. You may or may not grade the scheduling exercise (using Scheduling the Grading Form; Figure XIII: 2-C).

Alternatives and Variations:

Participants may complete the scheduling sheet prior to class. Class time can be used for discussion.

Concluding Points:

1. Scheduling is a complicated process requiring skill to work with detail as well as to view the larger perspective.

2. Scheduling requires more skill and practice than one critique can offer but this exercise can give the student an understanding of the process.

<u>Reading for Preparation</u>:

Cleland, V. (1982) Relating nursing staff quality to patients' needs.
    <u>Journal of Nursing Administration</u>, 12(4), 32.
Dale, R.L. and Mable, R.J. (1983) Nursing classification system:
    Foundation for personnel planning and control. <u>Journal of Nursing
    Administration</u>, 3(2), 10.

Figure XIII:2-A

Rationale for Answer Key

1.   Simmons -   1) Both weekends scheduled on are evenings.
                  2) Has requested holiday on 23rd but has already
                  been scheduled three-day WE (9th, 10th, 11th) per
                  request.

2.   Monroe   - Scheduled shifts appropriate, however, on the 22nd, she
                  makes second person on when only one is neededand on her off
                  day, the 23rd, there is not night coverage.

3.   Littleton- Prefers all nights in a stretch per request. Is scheduled
                  on eight odd shifts as 2 isolated days (13th and 14th) are
                  scheduled between her nights. Changing these days (13th and
                  14th) to nights not only gives her a stretch of nights but
                  also gives her a 50% rotation (10 nights).

4.   Jenkins - Prefers to work weekends or nights. Changing the WE of the
                  17th and 18th to nights not only provides night coverage,
                  but reduces the overstaffing on days. Granting the request
                  for nights on WE gives Jenkins 14 nights; so as she is not
                  needed on nights 13 and 14, placing her on days gives a more
                  reasonable number (12) of odd shifts.

5.   Hastings - Requested she can't work weekend evenings because of her
                  husband's bowling; however, generally everyone should work
                  one weekend of odd shift. Also, Hastings has only been
                  scheduled for four shifts the week of the 11th: scheduling
                  her evenings on the 14th corrects this overabundance of odd
                  shifts. Trade with Flynn on 15th.

6.   Jamison - Requested a "V" day with WE off to go out of town. Can
                  easily grant on 19th when she makes four on days.

7.   Boyd   - As Simmons' WE of third and fourth has been changed to days,
                  this leaves no evening coverage. Flynn has two WE's of
                  days. The third and fourth should be changed to evenings
                  giving her one WE of days and one WE of evenings. Changing
                  days on 15th to evenings still gives fair rotation and helps
                  Hastings' overabundance of evenings.

Rotation end up: D/E or D/N
D/E Simmons   11/9
D/N Monroe   9/11
D/N Littleton 10/10
D/N Jenkins   8/12, but wants both WE's nights
D/E Hastings   9/11
D/E Jamison   9/10 + 1 vacation day
D/E Boyd   8/9 + 3 class days
D/E Flynn   9/11

Figure XIII: 2-B

SCHEDULE ANSWER KEY

The schedule below is a proposed RN staff schedule for your medical division from the assistant head nurse. The RN's work either D/E or D/N rotations, 8-hour shifts, and optimally have 50% rotation. All RN's work off shifts one weekend a month except Ms. Jenkins who prefers to work nights each weekend she works. Ms. Littleton prefers to have her nights scheduled in a stretch. Minimum staffing is two on days, one on evenings, and one on nights on the weekends. Weekday minimums are two on days, two on evenings, and one on nights.

Please critique the schedule and make suggested changes in red pencil.

DATE	28	29	30	31	1	2	3	4	5	6	7	8	9	10	11	12	13	14	15	16	17	18	19	20	21	22	23	24	25	Nights or Evenings
STATUS	SUN	M	T	W	T	F	S	SUN	M	T	W	T	F	S	SUN	M	T	W	T	F	S	SUN	M	T	W	T	F	S	SUN	
J. Simmons — RN	X	D	D	D	D	X	X	D	D	E	E	E	E(R)	X(R)	X(R)	D	D	D	X	E	E	E	E	E	D	D	D	X	X	9
B. Monroe — RN	N	X	D	D	N	X	X	D	D	N	N	N	N	X	X	N	N	X	N	N	N	X	N	N	N	N	N	N	N	11
M. Littleton — RN	D	X	D	D	D	D	X	X	D	D	D	X	D	D	D	X	X	N	N	N	N	X	N	N	N	N	D	D	D	10
D. Jenkins — RN	X	N	N	N	X	N	N	N	N	X	N	N	N	D	X	D	D	X	D	D	D	X	D	D	D	D	D	X	D	12
E. Hastings — RN	X	E	E	E	D	X	X	D	D	D	E	X	E	E	X	D	D	D	X	E	E	E	E	E	E	E	E	X	X	11
F. Jamison — RN	D	D	D	X	D	D	D	X	D	D	D	X	X	D	D	D	X	X	D	D	D	X	E	E	E	X	X	D	D	10
S. Boyd — RN	E	X	C	D	D	X	X	D	D	C	D	X	E	C	E	X	X	D	D	X	E	E	E	E	E	X	E	E	D	10
M. Flynn — RN	X	E	E	E	X	E	E	X	E	E	E	E	E	E	X	X	D	D	X	D	D	X	D	D	D	D	D	X	X	11
Minimums:																														
2 Days	2	2	4	3	3	2	2	2	3	3	3	3	2	3	4	3	2	2	3	3	2	3	3	3	3	2	2			
1 Evenings	1	2	2	2	2	2	2	2	2	1	2	2	2	2	1	1	2	2	1	2	3	2	1	1						
1 Nights	1	1	1	1	2	1	1	2	1	1	1	1	1	1	1	1	2	1	1	1	1	1	1	1						

Would you grant the following requests?

A. Ms. Simmons has requested a day off on the 23rd to entertain out-of-town relatives.
___ Yes ___ No, Why _____

G. Ms. Boyd has requested to take a class in conflict resolution offered by the hospital's in-services department on the 31st, 7th, and 14th.
___ Yes ___ No, Why _____

F. Ms. Jamison has requested a vacation day with a weekend to give her 3 days off sometime during the month. She wants to go out of town to visit friends.
___ Yes ___ No, Why _____

E. Ms. Hastings has left you a message stating she cannot work weekend evenings because she can't get a regular babysitter and it's her husband's night to bowl.
___ Yes ___ No, Why _____

Figure XIII: 2-C

SCHEDULING GRADING FORM

Assess to determine if student has:

1.   Scheduled employees appropriate number of shifts.
        a)   Boyd has too many shifts during week of the 18th

2.   Provided minimum staffing for each day.
        a)   Put Jenkins on nights 17th and 18th.
        b)   Switch Monroe to off 22nd and to nights 23rd.

3.   Provided consistent staffing, i.e., do not schedule four on one day and two on next when it could easily be changed to three on each day. This is not vital but would be best.

4.   Honored employee preferences as much as possible.
        a)   Jenkins working nights each weekend she works.
        b)   Littleton scheduled for nights in a stretch.

5.   Given employees even number of shift rotations while maintaining consistent staffing. Some employees have more than 50% rotations.

6.   Equalized weekend rotations to off shifts.
        a)   Simmons should be changed to days on the third and fourth and either Flynn or Hastings to evenings on the third and fourth.

7.   Granted requests appropriately.
        a)   Simmons can be spared on the 23rd and have minimal staffing. It should be realized she requested and was granted a 3-day weekend the previous weekend.
        b)   Boyd can be granted request. Granting of this request demonstrates willingness to develop subordinates.

MODULE XIII: 3

Exercise: Handling complaints from Patients, Family Members and Staff

Objectives:

1.   To provide the opportunity to practice skills in handling complaints.

2.   To examine one's ability to remain nondefensive and deal with complaints directly.

Instructor's Role: To maintain triad role plays and lead large group discussion.

Operating Procedures, Hints and Cautions:

1.   This exercise will be more effective if participants use realistic situations and "get into" their parts.

2.   A discussion of active listening and nonverbal communication can facilitate this exercise. (See Chapter 4 of the textbook).

3.   Encourage observers to give feedback on nonverbal as well as verbal behavior. Participants can often say the appropriate words but nonverbally communicate defensively or angrily.

4.   Briefly review the key behaviors located in the Student Workbook (Module XIII:3) with participants before the role plays.

Alternatives and Variations:

You may want to role-play a situation with a class member as a demonstration for the entire class.

Concluding Points:

1.   Use of behavior modeling in this exercise may be helpful, i.e., to watch others "model" the appropriate behavior.

2.   Encourage role players to feel anger if possible. Then be sure to allow time to talk about angry feelings before students leave the class.

Reading for Preparation:

Katz, D. and Kahn, R. (1978) The Social Psychology of Organizations. New York: John C. Wiley & Sons.
Thompson, A.M. and Wood, M.D. (1980) Management Strategies for Women. New York: Simon & Schuster.

MODULE XIV: 1

Exercise: Dealing With Physicians

Objectives:

1. To increase understanding of the physician/nurse relationship.

2. To promote awareness of individual problems in dealing with physicians.

3. To provide an opportunity to practice dealing with physicians and to obtain group feedback.

Instructor's Role: To monitor triad role plays, encourage self-awareness, and lead large group discussion.

Operating Procedures, Hints, and Cautions:

1. Become familiar with information on assertiveness, conflict resolution, and physician/nurse relationships.

2. Read the corresponding exercise in the Student Workbook and complete the Physician Encounter Form for yourself.

3. Remember that participants will have a variety of experiences to share. Prevent this from becoming a complaint session by focusing on problem analysis and recognition of patterns in behavior, feelings and thoughts.

4. Be prepared to offer ideas for improving encounters with physicians to help participants clarify values and differentiate values from facts. For example, some participants may insist that physicians by nature want to give orders to nurses rather than ask for assistance. This is a value judgment. A fact may be that this participant has been given orders by several physicians in the past.

Alternatives and Variations:

A role play by two volunteers for the entire class may be useful. This would allow more discussion and better resolution of problems. However, some individual participants would not be able to practice. Determine which approach is best by considering the role-play experience of the students, their comfort level in the whole group, and the need for general discussion.

Concluding Points:

1. Physicians do have some common traits/behaviors as a group but, as individuals, their traits and behaviors vary.

2. Sexism has not been eliminated by the women's movement and

legislation.

3.   A woman's early socialization to be submissive with authority and with men and experiences in nursing contribute to the conflict between physicians and nurses.

4.   Continuing clear messages to staff on role expectations is a necessity for good nurse/physician relationships.

Reading for Preparation:

Bates, B. (1970) Doctor and nurse: Changing roles and relations. New England Journal of Medicine, 283, 129.

Johnston, P.F. (1983) Improving the nurse/physician relationship. The Journal of Nursing Administration. 13(3), 19-20.

Kerfoot, K. (1989) Nurse physician collaboration: a cost quality issue for the nurse manager. Nursing Economics 7, 335-338.

Nurse-physician-administrator Relationships. (Summer, 1983) Nursing Administration Quarterly, 7(4): entire issue

MODULE XIV: 2

Exercise: Dealing With Conflicts: Being the Mediator

Objectives:

1. To facilitate understanding of the methods of conflict resolution, particularly the collaborative method.

2. To provide practice in collaborative conflict resolution.

3. To obtain feedback from others on being the mediator.

Instructor's Role: To monitor the role plays and small group discussion.

Operating Procedures, Hints, and Cautions:

1. Be familiar with methods of conflict resolution and the collaborative approach.

2. Encourage participants to "get into" their roles and to not be compliant disputing parties. If members play their roles too cooperatively, there will be little challenge to the mediator.

3. Review the Evaluation Form in Module XIV:2 of the Student Workbook.

4. Remember that there will be four role plays that will take more time.

Alternatives and Variations:

1. Have participants think up their own situations but keep them to situations in which the disputing parties are equals.

2. Use this exercise with the behavior rehearsal technique and do only two role plays. This will encourage more adherence to the key behaviors and allow some participants to learn vicariously.

Concluding Points:

Collaborative problem solving doesn't always work. Here are the common pitfalls: not dealing with the emotions first, i.e., trying to negotiate before feelings are calmed; failing to adequately define the problem; not working out the specific details; judging during brainstorming; not following up; ignoring hidden agenda; and hurrying the process.

<u>Reading for Preparation</u>:

Bolten, R. (1979) <u>People Skills</u>. Prentice-Hall.
Brown, C.D. (1983) <u>Managing Conflict at Organizational Interfaces</u>. Reading,
    MA: Addison-Wesley.
Filley, C.A. (1975) <u>Interpersonal Conflict Resolution</u>, Glenview, IL:
    Scott, Foresman.
Gordon, T. and Burch, N. (1974) <u>Teacher Effectiveness Training</u>. New York:
    Peter H. Wyden.
King, D. (1981) Three cheers for conflict. <u>Personnel</u>, <u>58</u>:13.
Ruble, T. and Thomas, K. (1976) Support for a two-dimensional model of
    conflict behavior. <u>Organizational Behavior and Human Performance</u>,
    <u>16</u>:145

MODULE XIV: 3

Exercise: Managing Upward Communication: Dealing With Higher Administration

Objectives:

   1. To provide the opportunity to practice effective communication with superiors.

   2. To stimulate thinking about the importance of a good relationship with the boss.

   3. To obtain feedback from others on performance in taking a problem to the boss.

Instructor's Role: To monitor the triad role plays and lead large group discussion.

Operating Procedures, Hints, and Cautions:

   1. Be familiar with issues involved in upward communication.

   2. Read the Key Behaviors for Taking a Problem to the Boss and be able to clarify for the participants.

   3. Think of several role play situations to offer to participants if they ask for help.

   4. Encourage participants to assess any situation to determine the best tactic for use with the boss.

   5. Some participants may have negative experiences with bosses. Encourage them to take responsibility for their "half" of the relationship. This is difficult and some participants may be closed to new methods or may simply want validation that the boss was "impossible." Try to avoid this conclusion.

Alternatives and Variations:

   If the group size is approximately 3 to 15, use the behavioral rehearsal method. Participants learn a great deal from each other by watching the role play. Don't expect to do more than three role plays in 45 minutes.

Concluding Points:

   1. Upward communication involves nonverbal behavior as well as verbal. Tune in to your boss's nonverbal behaviors. This will help you find good timing for bringing up a new or debatable idea.

   2. Remember that the direct way is best; however, successful communication with a boss may require some power of influential tactics. For example, if you know your boss likes to feel like the "adviser," then give him/her the opportunity to advise you.

271

Accept it graciously and your boss will be more likely to accept your advice.

3. Women have special issues relating to upward communications in management, e.g., fear of being assertive or challenging with a boss, trying to please too much, or inattentiveness to the needs of the boss due to a lack of experience.

Reading for Preparation:

Filley, J.A.C. (1975) Interpersonal Conflict Resolution: Glenview, IL: Scott, Foresman.
Hegarty, C. (1980) How to Manage Your Boss. New York: Rawson, Wade Publisher.
Marriner, A. (1982) Managing Conflict, Nursing Management, 13:2931
Patton, B.R. and Giffin, K. (1981) Interpersonal Communication in Action. New York: Harper and Row.
St. John, W.D. (1983) Successful communications between supervisors and employees, Personnel Journal, 16, 5-9.

MODULE XIV: 4

Exercise: Handling Defensiveness in Yourself and Others

Objectives:

1. To increase awareness of the aspects of situations/persons that create defensiveness.

2. To provide the opportunity to practice dealing with defensiveness in others in realistic situations.

Instructor's Role: To monitor small group experience and triad role plays and serve as a resource for ideas.

Operating Procedures, Hints, and Cautions:

1. Be familiar with concepts of active listening and interpersonal communication skills.

2. When participants are in small groups, visit each group and offer ideas for reducing defensiveness.

3. Be prepared to assist participants in analysis of the Identifying Your Buttons Form to find patterns. Fill this form out for yourself and look for patterns in order to better help the participants.

Alternatives and Variations:

1. Participants can role-play in the large group rather than in triads. This will allow more group ideas to flow.

2. The Identifying Your Buttons Form can be discussed as a large group if participants are comfortable enough to share more personal feelings with the whole group.

Concluding Points:

1. Breathing and relaxation techniques can be very helpful in reducing tension during a defensive encounter.

2. Remember that a postponement of a discussion must be done carefully. Set a specific time/place and try to settle immediately if at all possible.

3. Reducing defensiveness is a process. Stick to active listening and with persistence, it will work in most cases.

<u>Reading for Preparation</u>:

Lange, A.J. and Jakubowski, P. (1976). <u>Responsible Assertive Behavior</u>.
    Champaign, IL: Research Press.
Osborn, S.M. and Harris, G.G. (1975) <u>Assertive Training for Women</u>.
    Springfield, IL: Charles C. Thomas Publisher.

MODULE XV: 1

Exercise: Assessing Productivity

ANSWERS

1. Unit XYZ Activity Report

MONTH	PATIENT DAYS	DIRECT CARE HOURS	TOTAL PAID PERSONNEL HOURS
JANUARY	464	3712	5568
FEBRUARY	483	3961	5942
MARCH	490	3871	5795
APRIL	455	3867	5812
MAY	421	3347	5028
JUNE	419	3350	5047
JULY	402	3216	5002
AUGUST	404	3302	5118
SEPTEMBER	439	3464	5092
OCTOBER	447	3621	5540
NOVEMBER	468	3884	5748
DECEMBER	470	3845	5729
TOTALS	5362	43440	65421
MEAN	446.8	3620	5451.8

2. 65421 total paid personnel hours x $15.00 per hour = $981,315

3. The completed deviation bar graph should look like the following:

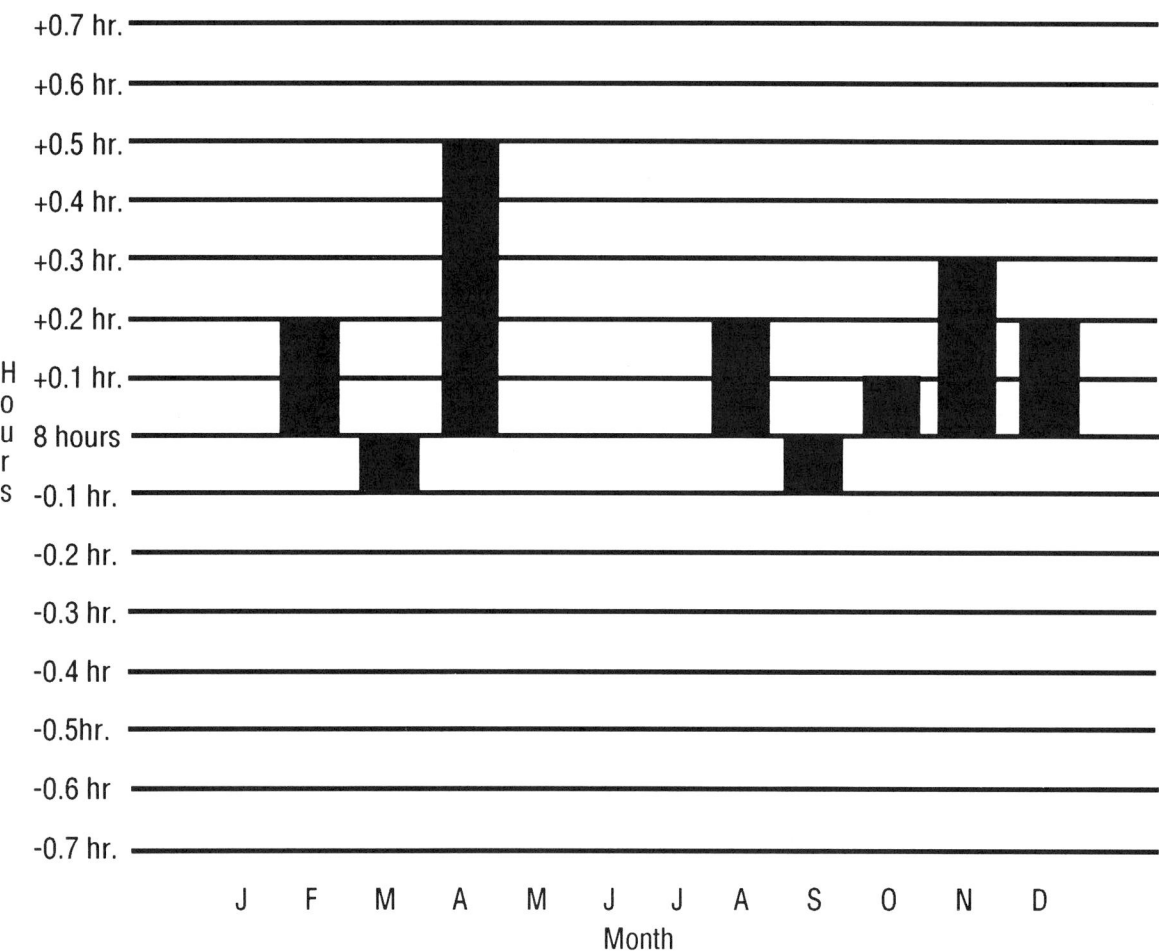

Seaside Hospital

Unit Performance Monitoring--January-June

Cost Center	Required YTD	Hours of Care Actual YTD	Variance	Pct. Prod.
General Surgery	2580	2702	- 122	95
General Medicine	3242	3291	49	99
Oncology	1693	1679	- 14	101
Neurology	2100	2089	11	101
Obstetrics	1814	1812	2	100
Gynecology	2631	2683	- 52	98
ICU	5796	6193	- 97	94
CCU	5361	6402	-1041	84
Telemetry	3787	4994	-1207	76
Orthopedics	2220	3530	-1310	63

2.   The assumption is that the required number of nursing hours can provide the quantity and quality of care the nursing unit desires to produce.

3.   There would be greatest concern about the CCU, Telemetry and Orthopedic units because each has a productivity percentage below 85%, which is the low point of the commonly used range of acceptable performance (i.e. 85% to 115%).

Exercise: Handling a Staff Member with Chemical Dependency

Objectives:

1.   To increase awareness of problems in addressing chemical
       dependency in nurses.

2.   To examine potential ways to intervene with a chemically dependent
       nurse and to consider the consequences of such actions.

3.   To improve attitudes toward nurses with problems of chemical
       dependence.

Instructor's Role: To facilitate group discussion of case.

Operating Procedures, Hints and Cautions:

1.   Familiarize yourself with the issues involved in intervening in
       cases of chemical dependency using the suggested readings.
       Particular attention is directed to Chemical Dependency in
       Nursing: The Deadly Diversion by Eleanor Sullivan, Bissell, and
       Williams (Addison-Wesley, 1988).

2.   Read the case and discussion questions before class. Formulate
       your own answers.

Case Discussion

Marie must intervene in this case. She has an excellent clinician in
Joan and will be worried about replacing such a valued employee, but she
cannot let the situation continue.

First, she should seek the assistance of her supervisor and, if
available, an employee assistance counselor or treatment center staff in
planning an intervention. The goal of intervention is to get the person to
treatment to be evaluated for a possible problem with chemical abuse.
Resource people can help Marie prepare for the intervention with Joan. Next,
she should collect all the data she can on objective indicators of a problem
(e.g., narcotics records, patient records, observed changes in Joan's
appearance or performance). Also she needs to plan where to refer Joan for
evaluation of the problem and decide what her actions will be if Joan does not
agree to go. Finally, she should decide when to do an intervention and who
should attend.

One possible scenario would be the following. Marie collects the
information she needs to present Joan with data and has talked with a local
treatment center that is prepared to accept Joan immediately into treatment.
Also, Marie has checked with the hospital's benefit's office and knows that
Joan's health insurance will pay her treatment costs. She calls Joan into her

office early in the morning. Her supervisor agrees to participate.

Joan is surprised to be confronted with the information and begins to explain that she has been taking medications for sleep and for migraine headaches and that it was all prescribed. She explains that she has had to waste excessive amounts of narcotics because the fast pace of the unit makes her try to move too quickly and make mistakes. When confronted with the altered records, however, Joan breaks down and starts to cry, saying she's been trying so hard to be a "good nurse" that she has taken the drugs to "feel better and work harder". Marie assures her that she is a "good nurse" and that, in fact, the majority of nurses who get into trouble with alcohol or drugs are those who are very successful in nursing and that most of them recover and return to nursing. The supervisor further assures Joan that the hospital will have a job for her when she completes treatment although she may have to transfer to another unit for a period of time. A friend of Joan's is called to drive her to the treatment center.*

Marie does not need to report Joan to the state board of nursing if she is assured of Joan's continuing recovery. Recovery is monitored in various ways but most commonly by a return-to-work contract specifying what the nurse will do to ensure recovery for a one to two year period. (See Chapter 8 of the textbook for an example of a return-to-work contract.) Usually these behaviors include attendance at Alcoholics Anonymous, participation in follow-up care at a treatment center and, usually, random urine screens for drugs. The contract also spells out the consequences if the nurse does not meet the behaviors specified or returns to alcohol or other drug use. Possible consequences could include re-evaluation by treatment counselor and subsequent return to treatment, dismissal from the job, and report to the State Board of Nursing.

After the conference, Marie needs to write a report on what occurred, agreed to behaviors and contingencies.

*The above story is true with only the names changed.

MODULE XV: 3

Exercise: Managing the Change Process

Objectives:

1. To learn how to diagnose the forces of change.

2. To practice overcoming resistance to change through planning.

Instructor's Role: To give directions for the small group experience and to monitor small group feedback and discussion.

Operating Procedures, Hints, and Cautions:

1. Be familiar with the change process and the model of Lewin presented in the text.

2. Make sure students think about an organizational situation that needs change before class.

3. Review Forms I and II before class.

4. Change is often resisted and sometimes actively opposed. One way to overcome resistance and its negative effects is to get employees involved in planning the change so that it does not seem so unfamiliar and threatening to them. Before talking with an employee, try to determine what is in it for employees affected by the change.
   a. Explain the general situation and <u>why</u> a change is necessary.
   b. Explain the details and problems of the change and discuss <u>how it will affect the employee</u>.
   c. <u>Ask the employee for his help</u>.
   d. Ask the employee to think about ways to implement the change and schedule a follow-up discussion.

5. <u>Some Additional Thoughts</u>.
   a. Give advance notice of change. Get negative reactions out of the way prior to actual implementation.
   b. Explaining "why" is critical.
   c. Our schools teach young people to ask "why".
   d. Tell employee <u>what's in it for him/her</u>.
   e. Give change a <u>positive</u> rather than problem orientation.
   f. If we don't explain the change, someone else will, and the reasons could be all or partly wrong.
   g. When someone else explains why, it brings attention, status, recognition, and leadership, for example, to that person instead of the supervisor.
   h. Caution! Information is power. Be careful about talking to one person.

Alternatives and Variations:

This exercise can be done as a take home written exercise. Group discussion of results can be done or not, as you wish.

Concluding Points:

Discuss the importance of the change process in nursing and health care today. Discuss the use of the different models of change. Also, discuss the implications of change.

Reading for Preparation:

Hoffer, A. (1986) Facilitating Change: choosing the appropriate strategy, Journal of Nursing Administration 16:18-22.
Lipcott, G.C., Longseth, P. and Mossge, J. (1985) Implementing Organizational Change. San Francisco: Jossey-Bass.

Exercise: Critiquing Research

The following article and student handout are provided for assistance in assigning a research critique project. We highly recommend Mary Castles' book, A Primer of Nursing Research, (1987, Saunders) for review in such an activity.

Priming Students to Read Research Critically

Robert P. Heaney
M. Janet Barger-Lux

Health professionals conduct and present research in order to change the way health care is practiced. For practitioners either to adopt or reject the changes that findings suggest, they must be able to evaluate the research. We designed the undergraduate research course at Creighton University's School of Nursing to teach them to do just that. The course, which we created specifically for professional consumers of research, is multiprofessional, both in the students it serves and in the kinds of research with which it deals.

We became involved in designing this course in 1978, when the dean of the nursing school asked for a multiprofessional consultation on the senior-level research course. The content of that course had varied from year to year, depending on who taught it. At the time, Creighton was conducting an all-health-sciences project in computer-supported curriculum design, intended, among other things, to determine commonalities among the health professions curricula [1]. The course was part of that project.

The task force set up to analyze needs included representatives from nursing, pharmacy, allied health, and medicine, but their primary focus was on nursing since, of all the health professions programs on campus, only the nursing school already offered a research course. The task force started by looking at what the nursing faculty wanted its students to learn about research. It soon became clear that they did not intend to teach students to do research —how to plan, organize, complete, and publish it, or even to know how researchers do these things. The baccalaureate program is designed to prepare individuals to practice professional nursing. Although some graduates go on to graduate study and ultimately do research, most do not, and the committee's nursing representatives thought it would be inappropriate to require individuals preparing to begin professional nursing practice to know how to do research. Instead, the faculty wanted graduates to be able to read research critically and to react intelligently to it, changing their professional practices when the evidence warrants it and rejecting change when the evidence is insufficient.

The task force next had to determine how to achieve this goal without retracing the steps of research. Committee members agreed that the skills required to evaluate research critically are distinct from the skills required to do it, just as the skills needed to understand and appreciate music differ from those needed to compose or perform it.

If researchers alone could understand research, most of us would have to accept their conclusions without question.

Textbooks offered us little help. Although many of the major nursing research texts on the market then had been written for undergraduates, they tended to be "how to" books—not how to evaluate, but how to perform. The tables of contents told the story, listing chapters on "Selecting a Problem," "Searching the Literature," "Research Planning," "Framing the Hypotheses," "How to Apply for Grant Support," "Instruments for Data Collection," and "Publication of the Research report." Few of the texts we reviewed included information on evaluating research outcomes, investigative design, what can go wrong, principal pitfalls, or problems corresponding to the types of research.

The medical texts were no better. Most were dominated by epidemiology and statistics, emphasizing how to do those things, not how to evaluate others' work. Although Mainland's *Elementary Medical Statistics* does contain appropriate material, it is not well organized for the course we envisioned, and it is out of print.

We decided next to use an analytical, highly structured curriculum design process then being put in place throughout the health sciences programs. The process involved systematically determining the elements in each instructional objective, from the most general to the most minute. We arrived at a structural design for the new course, choosing as its overall goal "to enable the student to interact in a professional manner with ongoing health-related research." The general goal contained three major elements: problem-solving in a context of variability; critical reading of the research literature; and ethical dimensions of human investigation. The design process also allowed us to specify instructional objectives related to each element, which we wrote into subgoals, as well as the logical relationship among their component elements. We eventually drafted more than 30 pages of hierarchically organized, logically connected instructional objectives. Figure 1 shows the top three levels as well as their major connections.

The objectives related to the ethical dimensions of human investigation are integral to achieving the overall course goal. As we developed them, we asked for input from members of the philosophy department, and we emphasized aspects of research that touch the millieu of entry-level health professionals. With these objectives, the course expands the concept of the responsible consumer of research to include the responsible colleague of researchers and the responsible advocate of research subjects. What we call the research perspective—an understanding of conclusion-drawing from experiences with situations that vary— underpins all three roles, even the ethical one. This conclusion follows from the realization that a study that involves human subjects cannot be morally defensible if it is not also scientifically sound. Researchers should not subject individuals to risk, or even to inconvenience, if, because of flawed design, a study cannot yield useful knowledge.

The entire set of instructional objectives constituted a detailed plan for teaching and for learning designed to equip entry-level professional nurses with skills for interpreting and reacting to the research literature and for interacting with research intelligently and ethically.

In translating the plan into an actual course, we decided to use lectures, reading assignments, and videotaped instruction [2]. The course occupies a full semester and carries two semester hours of academic credit. From the beginning, we incorporated two requirements: a series of practical exercises to bring about an understanding of variation and probability; and the structured evaluation of a published research report. For the first, each student must work out frequency distributions experientially, using disc sampling, card shuffling and dealing, and coin flipping and die throwing. The experiences become concrete bases for understanding the three fundamental probability analogies on which all statistical inferences are based. Accurate probabilistic thinking seems counter-intuitive, and we decided that hands-on experience with the variability produced by random chance alone would be a useful adjunct

Figure 1. Structural relationship of the top-most goals for the Creighton Nursing course on research

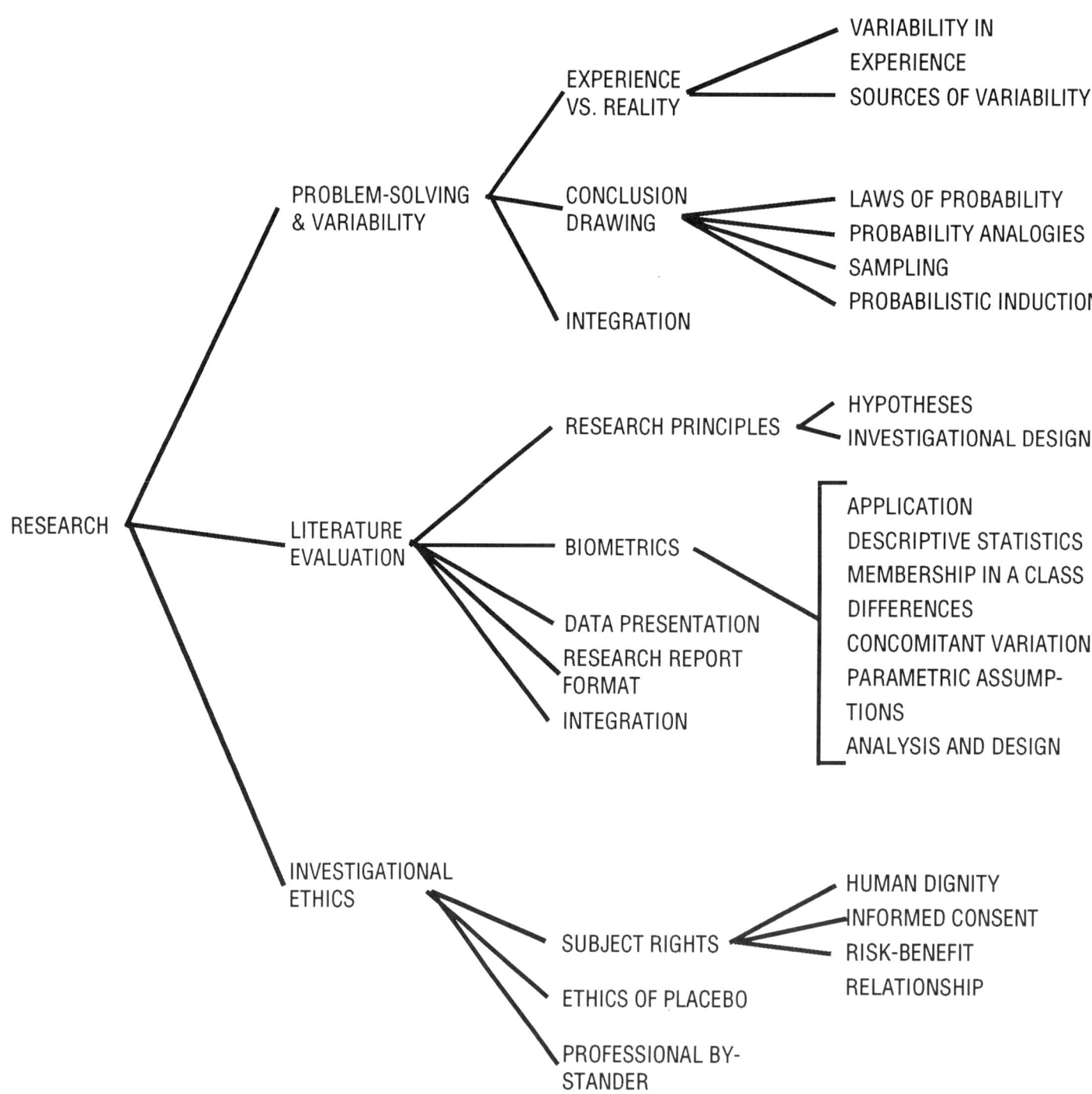

to the didactic treatment of conclusion-drawing from experiences subject to variation. [3].

The second requirement is for students to evaluate a published research report, first analyzing its structure, and design features and then critiquing it. A large library of articles from across the health-related disciplines allows us to avoid within-class duplication of assignments. The literature evaluation assignment follows classroom exercises in working through many examples of the same approach and process. The students tend to follow these classroom analyses easily, but using such skills independently is more difficult. Since being able to be intelligent professional consumers of research is the purpose of the course, we thought it was crucial to give the students an opportunity to try out these important new skills. The assignment occurs late in the course, after we have thoroughly covered investigative design, and we derive 40 percent of the final course grade for nursing students from performance on this paper.

The course design is cumulative—each part builds on, presumes, and uses everything that has gone before. For this reason, we adopted a grading system heavily weighted toward performance at the end of the course. We have observed more than a few students who, after being in a fog for several weeks, suddenly see how it all fits together.

Multiprofessional Approach

Early attention to research placed the nursing school in a position of leadership among the Creighton health professions programs. As the other faculties came to address the place of research in their own curricula, they looked at what nursing had already defined and found that, for the most part, the nursing objectives fit their own needs. For several years, the pharmacy school had offered a required mini-course called Literature Evaluation. When pharmacy faculty members examined the nursing plan for Research, they found that its objectives described exactly what they were trying to accomplish in their own course. The pharmacy school enthusiastically adopted the nursing plan of instruction, and pharmacy students were among the first to take the course together with nursing students.

Several of the allied health programs soon followed suit. The schools of medicine and dentistry adopted the nursing school's course goals as their own, making only minor wording changes. The pharmacy department's doctoral program had to add several objectives dealing with statistical computations, but members of the faculty were able to include this component in a few hours of instruction. Other program-specific differences were equally easy to accommodate. For example, different programs place different weights on the assigned paper, but this affects only the

calculation of the course grade, not the content or process of the course itself.

As more health profession programs have bought into the course, logistical problems such as scheduling and class size have prohibited a large-scale, interdisciplinary course. Also, the several student groups have different attitudes and tend to learn differently, and we found it difficult to respond to these differences in a large group setting. However, we have seen no appreciable difference in the level of readiness for the course between, for example, freshmen medical students and senior nursing students—which are to levels at which we teach the course. Eight years of experience support our conclusion that nursing students perform at least as well in this course as do the other student groups. Finally, we have judged that the experience of multiprofessional learning is valuable, and that it is important for health professional who will occupy varying positions on the power spectrum to experience parity as they wrestle with this course.

The multidesciplinary applicability of the nursing research objectives demonstrated that the skills required for evaluating professional research literature are common to all the health professions. It also put nursing in a position of leadership among the health profession programs, which was not only good for nursing, but also for the other schools and programs.

Another multiprofessional characteristic of the course is the material we teach students to evaluate. In the early stages of designing the course, we decided that our graduates should be able to react to the broad scope of health research, and that to gear the course to a single subset of the research would not allow students to meet the course goal. The various health professions cannot function in isolation—what the members of each profession do in their day-to-day work is influenced by advances in all professions. Therefore, to look at one subset of professional research would be too restricting. We also recognized that many research communications do not reach practitioners through their professional literature, but rather through the daily press and weekly news magazines. Many wire service reporters and science writers can capture the essential features of the structure and outcomes of investigations, and news stories abstracted from professional publications appear in the press daily. Patients and their families read these articles avidly, but, for the most part, they are not equipped to understand or to evaluate what they read. As nurses strive to answer patients' questions, they must be able to react professionally to the things their clients read. For this reason also, to have focused on only nursing research would have been inappropriately narrow.

Critical Thinking

The research course is rigorous, and it quickly acquired a reputation among the students as difficult. Although our expectations in terms of the depth of content are modest, students cannot do well simply by being able to recognize or recall items from a body of facts. In order to meet the course goal, they must be able to evaluate unfamiliar research reports, which requires an ability to think inductively—to examine the particular and find the general implied by it—and to use analogies. Students come to the course with varying abilities for inductive thinking. Some have poorly developed abilities in this area, and we constantly strive to find and use more effective teaching strategies to support the exercise of these intellectual skills.

Three years after we began to reconfigure our approach to teaching research to nursing students, the American Nurses' Association (ANA) promulgated a goal nearly identical to our own in its guidelines for research activities appropriate for a BSN graduate, who "reads, interprets, and evaluates research for applicability to nursing practice [4]." As it turned out, our course is broader in compass than the later ANA guideline, but in keeping with its spirit.

Robert P. Heaney, MD, is John A. Creighton University Professor at Creighton University in Omaha, Nebraska. M. Janet Barger-Lux, MS, is the director of professional services in the School of Nursing there.

From Nursing & Health Care, October, 1986, pp. 421-424. Reprinted with permission.

References

1. The Total-System Design (TSD) Project, undertaken in 1975 at Creighton University with funding from the W.K. Kellogg Foundation, involved the application of artificial intelligence technology to the design of instruction, with the resulting information used to support a computer-based health professions consultant, the COMMES system.

2. Heaney, Robert P., and Dougherty. Charles J., Research for Health Professionals: Design, Analysis, and Ethics, Ames: Iowa State University Press, in press.

3. Weaver, Warren, Lady Luck, The Theory of Probability, New York: Dover Publications, Inc., 1982.

4. American Nurses' Association Commission on Nursing Research. Guidelines for the investigative function of nurses, Kansas City: ANA, 1981.

Writing a Critique of a Research Paper

I. <u>Summary</u>-Describe in a few sentences the author's (a) conceptualization, (b) procedures, and (c) results. Confine yourself here only to what is important under each of the headings. If the author's abstract is well written, he or she may already have done this job for you.

II. <u>Critique</u> - Deal with the adequacy of conceptualization, procedures, and results in that order - preferably using numbered paragraphs to separate distinct criticisms. (Headings, such as the ones in this guide, typically are not employed.) Since it is useful for an author to have feedback about what is good in his or her paper, do not confine comments to negative ones if there is any merit in the manuscript. The following major points should be addressed in most instances.

   A. Conceptualization
      1. How well worked out is the author's conceptual framework for the study?
      2. Have alternative conceptualizations been acknowledged?
      3. Has there been adequate consideration of previous empirical findings relevant to the author's conceptualization or to important alternative conceptual frameworks?

   B. Procedures
      1. Do the research procedures relate satisfactorily to the conceptualization? That is, were independent and dependent variables well operationalized? (The author may have helped you here by providing manipulation checks.)
      2. Has the experiment been carefully conducted (particularly, has the author been on guard for potential sources of artifact in the data?) (No comment on this is necessary unless there are grounds for criticism.)
      3. Is the design adequate to test the author's hypothesis and are necessary control conditions included? (Controls are not necessary for all hypothesis tests.)

   C. Results and Discussion
      1. Have analyses appropriate to the design been properly employed?
      2. Have possible alternative interpretations been considered?
      3. If alternative interpretations have been rejected, has this been done on the basis of adequate data or compelling logic (e.g., procedures)?

   D. General
      1. Are there problems in writing style or organization?
      2. Is the research a significant contribution to the field?
      3. Determine the degree to which the article:
         a. meets its intended purpose
         b. is relevant to problems of which you are aware

Writing Instructions for a Written Critique

1.   The first section of the analysis should be a short description of the article and the purpose of the article. Do not make this section more than one-half page in length. Title this section, "Introduction."

2.   The second portion of the analysis should concentrate on questions raised in parts 2 and 3 of the reading instructions above. Title this section, "Selected Comments."
      (a)   The first subsection should contain a precise description of the problems encountered. (Reference every problem found to a particular line or paragraph of the article analyzed.) Title this subsection, "Troublesome Terms and Arguments."
      (b)   The second subsection should contain your approach to the problems you have raised and should be based on parts 3b and 3c of the reading instruction. This subsection should be titled, "Consideration of Problems."

3.   In the third section of the analysis, questions raised in your mind but not answered in the article should be stated, and the reasons the questions are worth answering should be explored. This section should be titled, "Additional Research."

4.   The fourth section should be a set of questions the reader should be capable of answering after having read the original article and your analysis. Title this section, "Questions."

NOTE: The purpose of this approach is not to debunk existing scholars, and you do not have license to lampoon or lambast what has been written by scholars. The purpose of this approach is to foster a critical understanding and a willingness to straighten out inconsistencies. Anyone who reads conscientiously will undoubtedly raise questions, and these honest questions are legitimate sources for the analysis you prepare.

5.   In writing an analysis, follow these writing habits:
      (a)   Organize the paper in the format described above.
      (b)   Connect paragraphs so that one paragraph flows smoothly from the preceding paragraph.
      (c)   Write precisely and avoid unnecessary adjectives.
      (d)   Avoid personal pronouns such as I, we, our, etc.
      (e)   Reference pages and paragraphs in the article analyzed in the following way: Following the sentence in which the reference is made, place in parentheses the page number and paragraph number of the item referred to. For example: The author introduces, but leaves undefined, the term, "Valence" (pg. 3, paragraph 4).

6.   Ask these questions of each sentence written in your own analysis:
      (a)   What does the sentence mean?
      (b)   Why is it true?
      (c)   What terms have been left undefined?

      (d)   What assumptions are unstated?
      (e)   What arguments are not complete?

If questions 6a and 6b cannot be answered, then the analysis should be reworked until they are answered. If you assume the undefined terms would be clear to another reader, then these terms should be left undefined. However, if the undefined terms may be ambiguous, you should clear up the ambiguity. For unstated assumptions, state that they are assumptions. For incomplete arguments, attempt to complete the argument or state why and where the argument is incomplete.

TRANSPARENCY MASTERS

2.1   THE HEALTH CARE INSTITUTION AS AN OPEN SYSTEM

2.2   TYPICAL BUREAUCRATIC STRUCTURE WITH SPECIAL FOCUS ON THE NURSING DEPARTMENT

2.8   DECENTRALIZED NURSING SERVICE

3.1   FACTORS AFFECTING THE NURSE MANAGER

5.1   NURSING PRODUCTIVITY FRAMEWORK

7.1   THE SHANNON-WEAVER COMMUNICATION MODEL

7.5   COMMUNICATION CHANNELS

8.2   INTEGRATED MODEL OF THE MOTIVATIONAL PROCESS

9.3   USE OF PARTICIPATIVE LEADERSHIP STYLES

10.1   STRESS BALANCE

14.2   REINFORCEMENT PROCESS

14.3   SOCIAL LEARNING THEORY

14.4   A MODEL OF THE EDUCATIONAL RELAPSE PROCESS

17.1   A DIAGNOSTIC MODEL OF EMPLOYEE ATTENDANCE

17.2   A MODEL OF VOLUNTARY EMPLOYEE TURNOVER

20.1   LEWIN'S FORCE-FIELD MODEL OF CHANGE

20.2   COMPARISON OF CHANGE MODELS

20.3   SEVEN STEPS OF PLANNED CHANGE: AN EXTENSION OF THE NURSING PROCESS

21.1   RISK MANAGEMENT ORGANIZATIONAL MODEL

22.1   CONFLICT PROCESS

THE HEALTH CARE INSTITUTION AS AN OPEN SYSTEM (Figure 2-1)

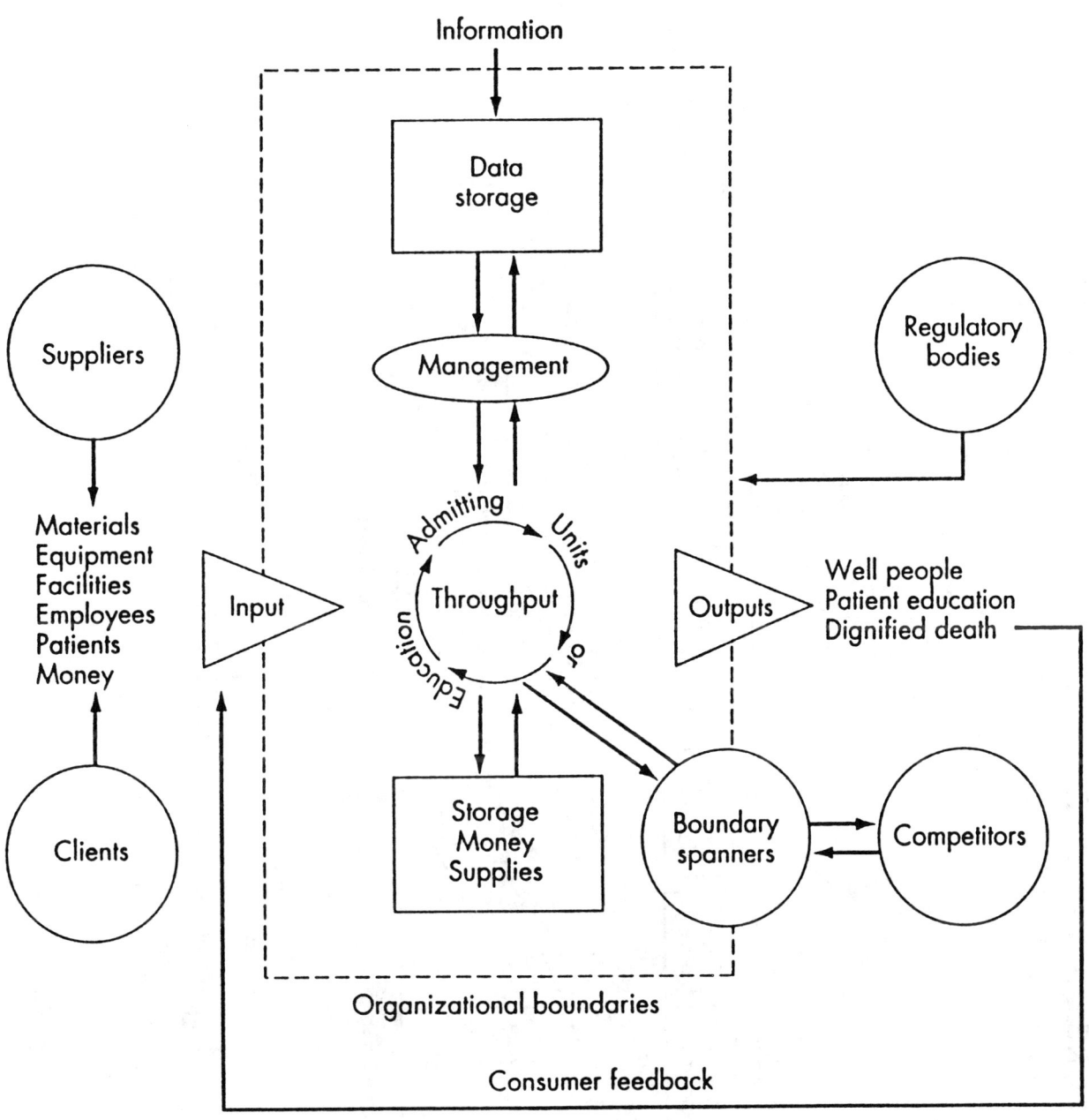

TYPICAL BUREAUCRATIC STRUCTURE WITH SPECIAL FOCUS ON THE
NURSING DEPARTMENT (Figure 2-2)

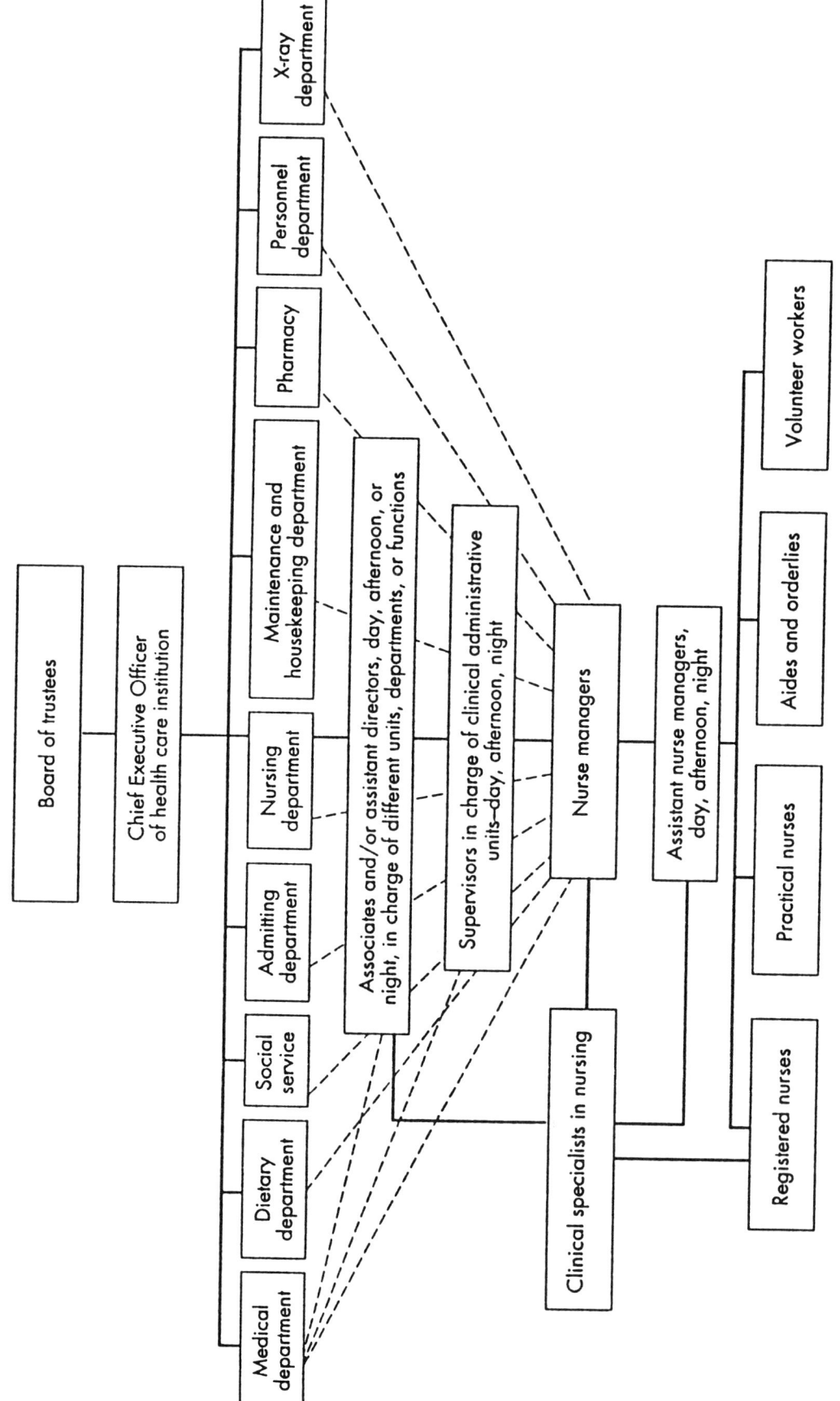

Copyright © Addison-Wesley Nursing

DECENTRALIZED NURSING SERVICE (Figure 2-8)

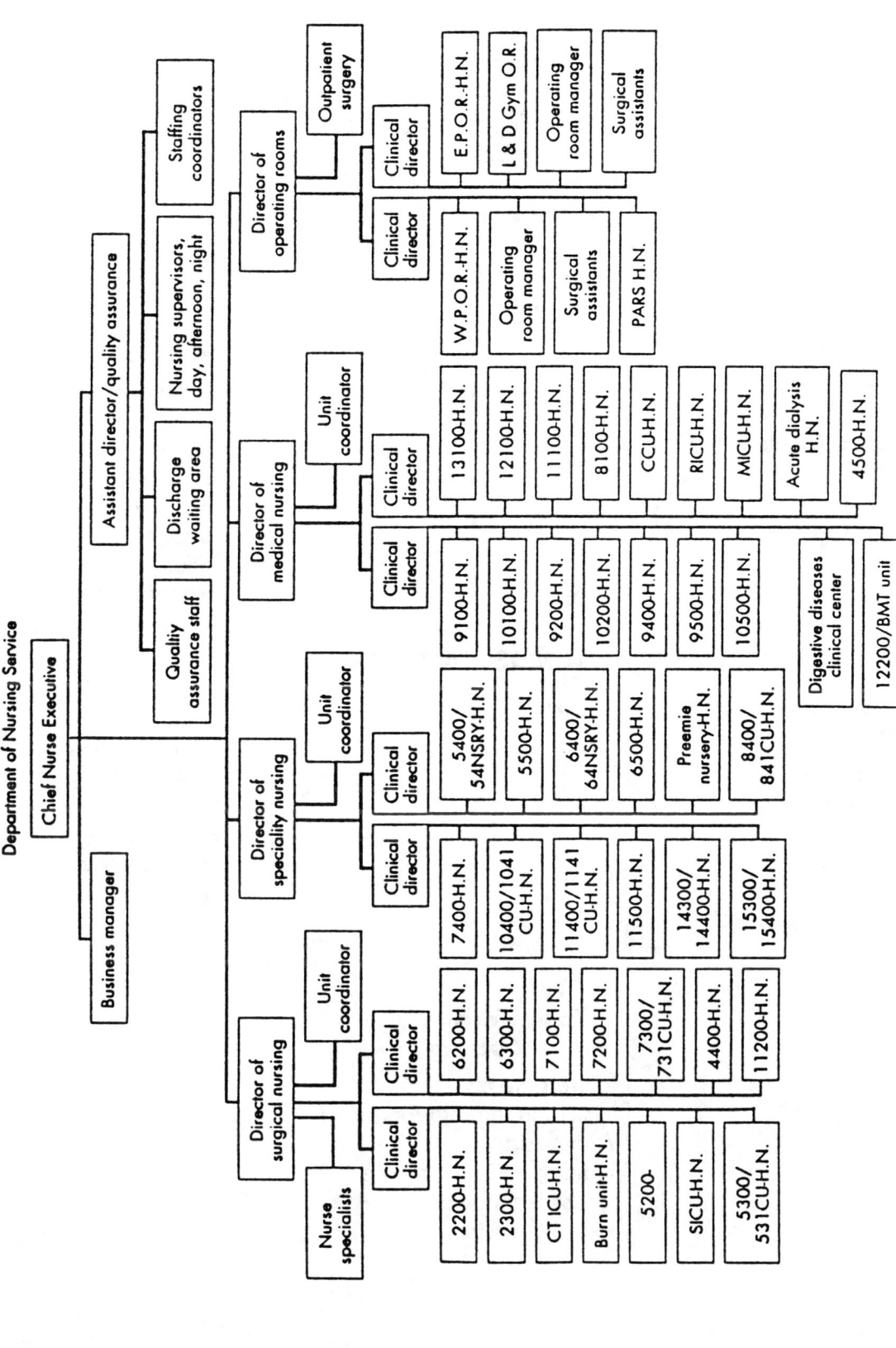

FACTORS AFFECTING THE NURSE MANAGER (Figure 3-1)

**Institutional
Structure**

Authority structure
Means of departmentalization
Span of control
Centralization vs. decentralization
Integrative systems
Control and measurement system
Recruitment and selection system
Reward system

**Environmental
Factors**

Economic
Legal/governmental
Market/competetive
Technological
Social/personnel

Work Social Structure

Institutional culture
Norms/sentiments/beliefs
Rituals
Language
Socialization processes
Roles/role conflict
Status system
Organizational climate

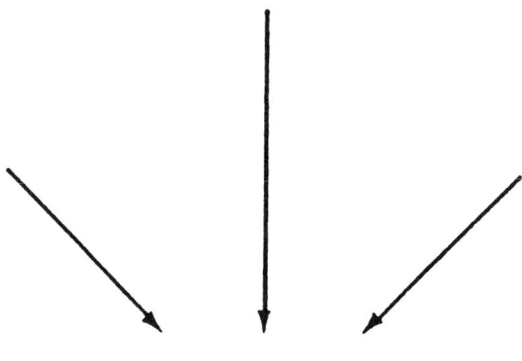

NURSE MANAGER

**Institutional
Objectives**

Product/service
Productivity/efficiency
Social
Human resource
Goal displacement
Participation in goal setting

People

Values/assumptions
Background
Status
Motivation
Learning style
Group processes/cohesiveness

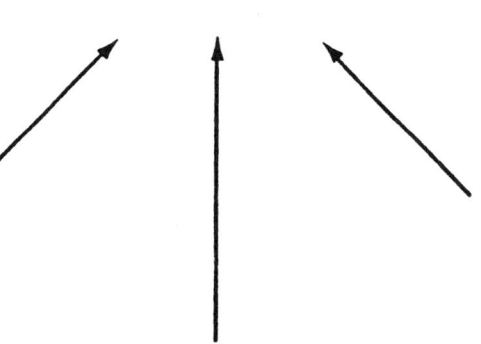

**Task/Technology
Factors**

Nature of tasks
Physical layout of workplace
Work design
Medical/nursing science
Process technology
Computer system

NURSING PRODUCTIVITY FRAMEWORK (Figure 5-1)

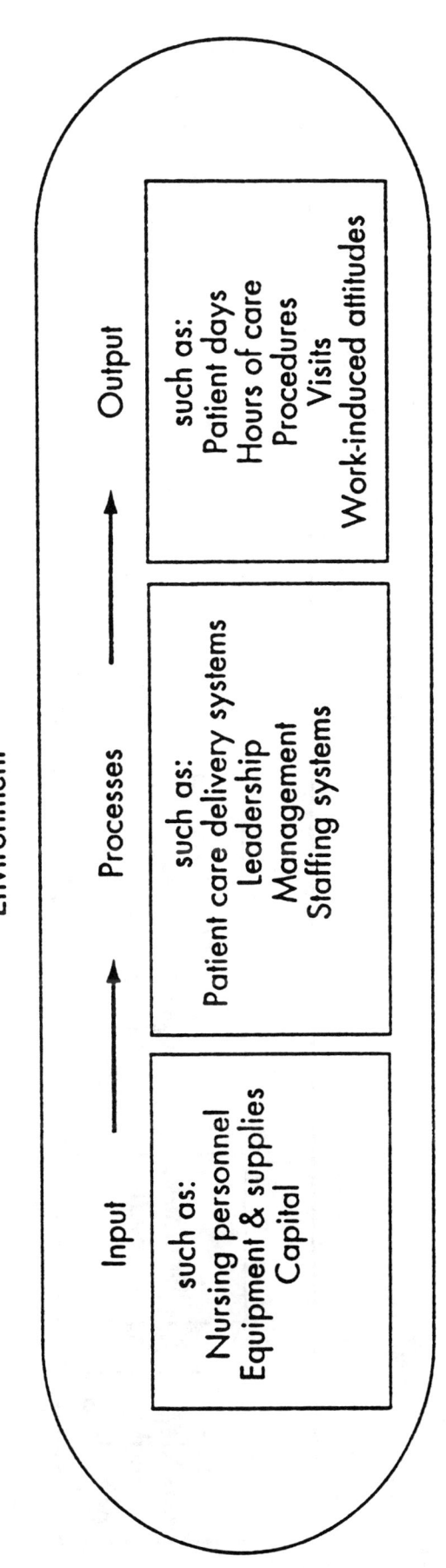

Environment

Input → Processes → Output

such as:
Nursing personnel
Equipment & supplies
Capital

such as:
Patient care delivery systems
Leadership
Management
Staffing systems

such as:
Patient days
Hours of care
Procedures
Visits
Work-induced attitudes

THE SHANNON-WEAVER COMMUNICATION MODEL   (Figure 7-1)

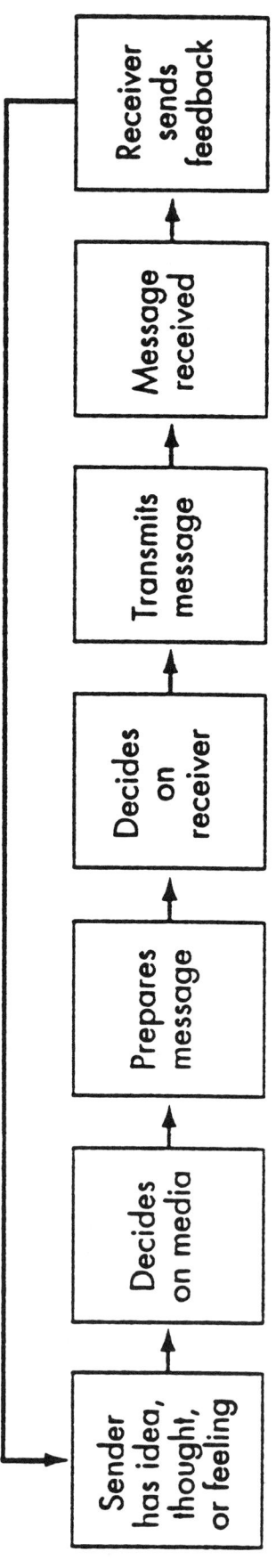

COMMUNICATION CHANNELS (Figure 7-5)

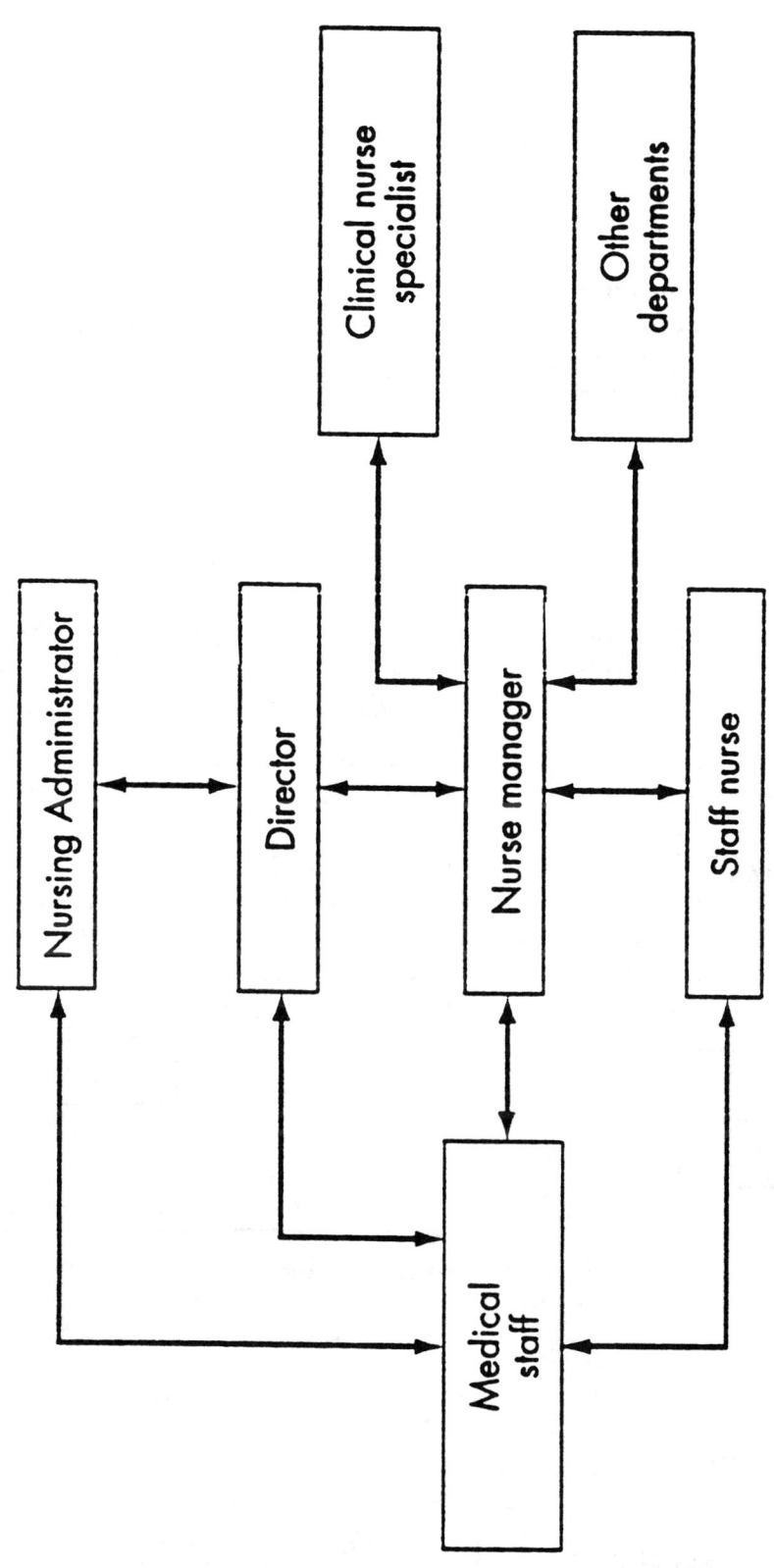

INTEGRATED MODEL OF THE MOTIVATIONAL PROCESS (Figure 8-2)

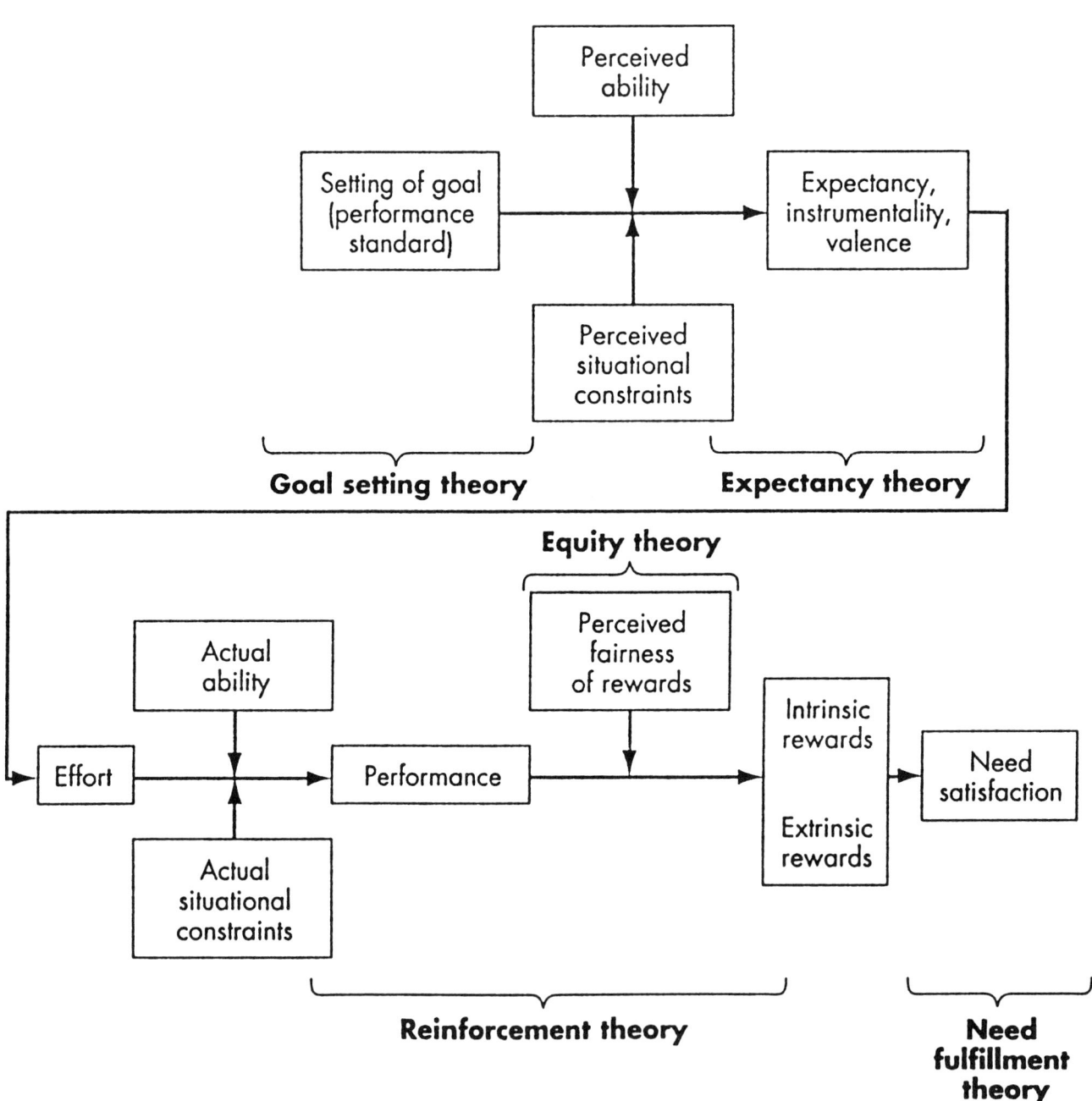

USE OF PARTICIPATIVE LEADERSHIP STYLES (Figure 9-3)

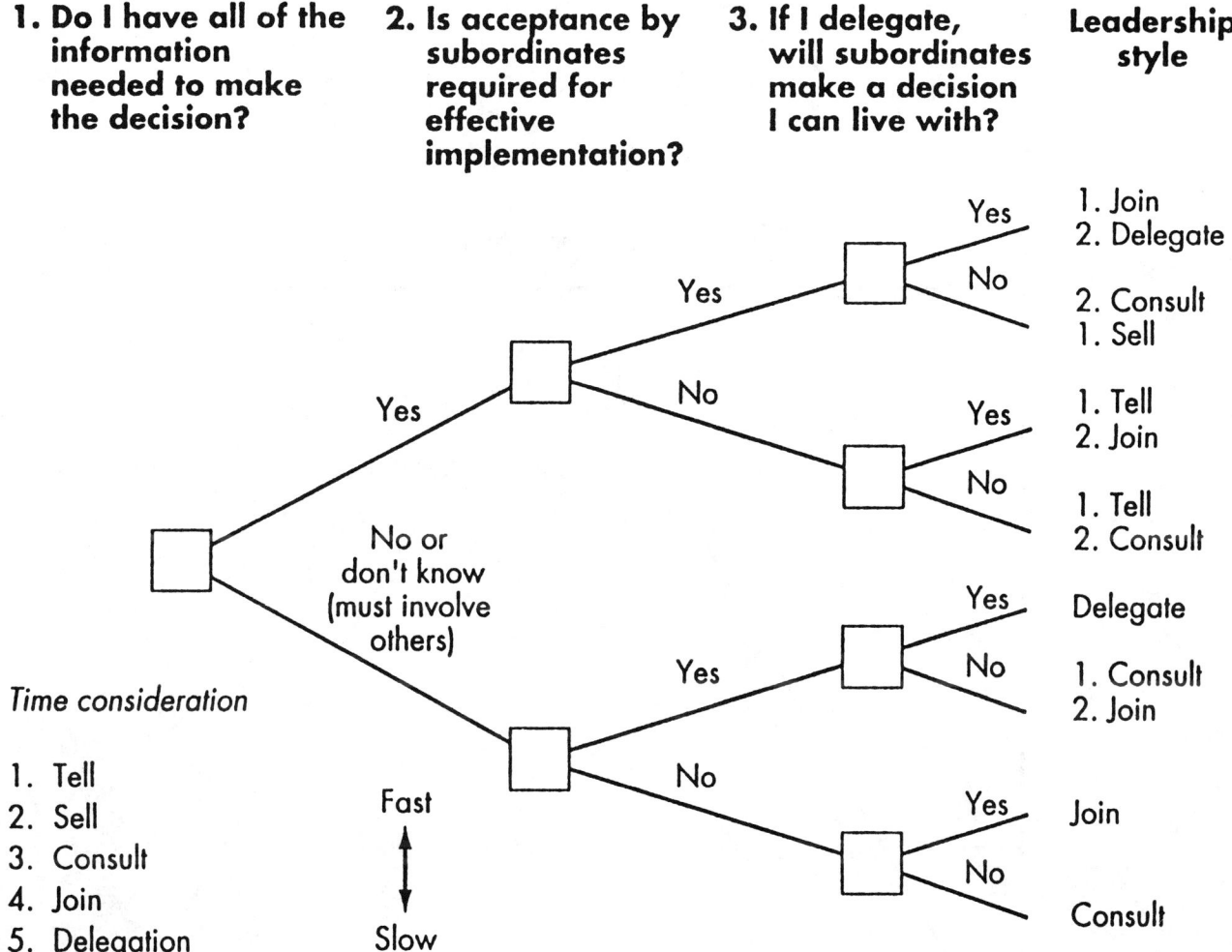

1. Do I have all of the information needed to make the decision?

2. Is acceptance by subordinates required for effective implementation?

3. If I delegate, will subordinates make a decision I can live with?

Leadership style

Yes
Yes
1. Join
2. Delegate

No
2. Consult
1. Sell

Yes

No
Yes
1. Tell
2. Join

No
1. Tell
2. Consult

Yes

No or don't know (must involve others)

Yes
Yes
Delegate

No
1. Consult
2. Join

No
Yes
Join

No
Consult

Time consideration

1. Tell
2. Sell
3. Consult
4. Join
5. Delegation

Fast
↕
Slow

STRESS BALANCE (Figure 10-1)

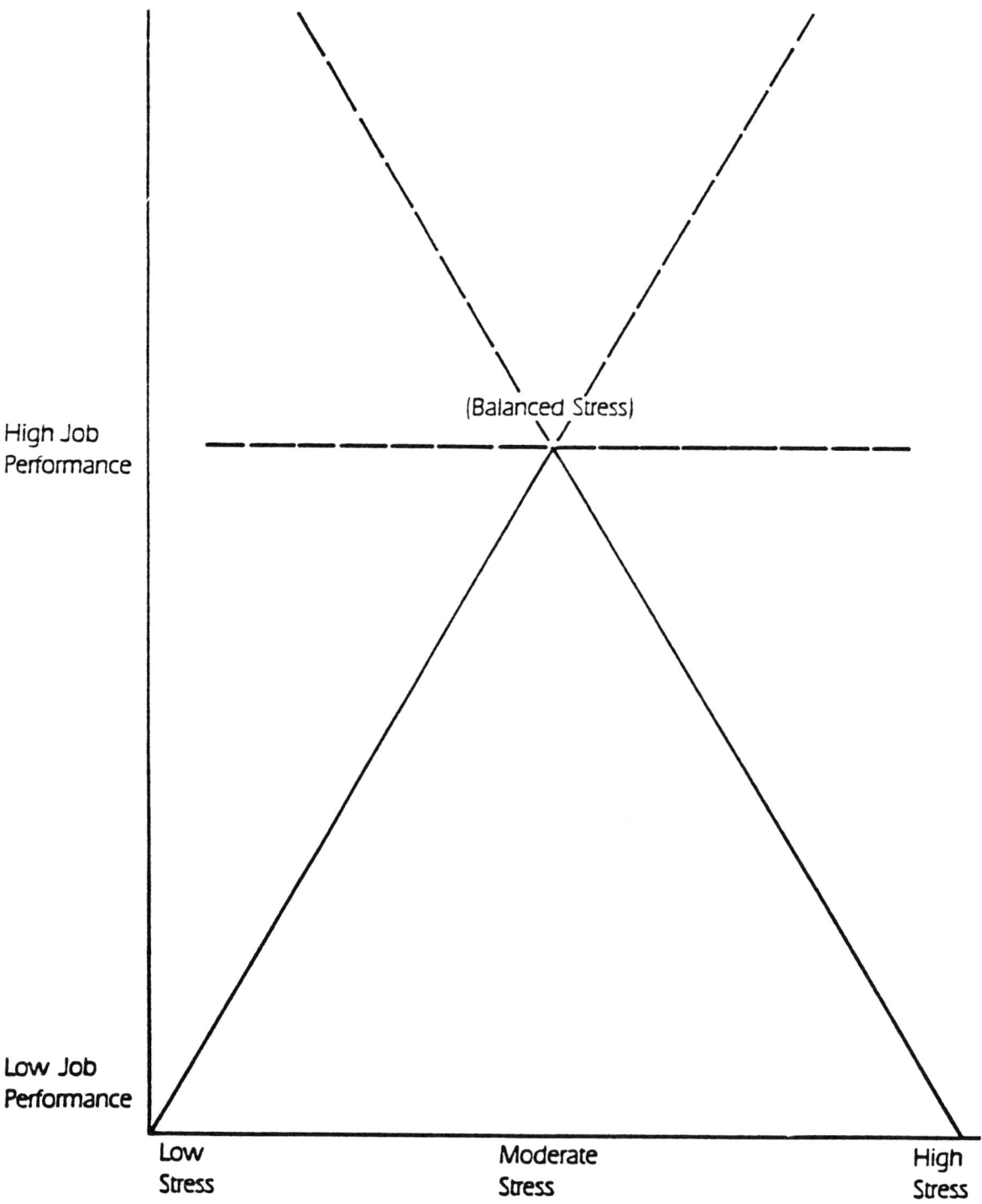

REINFORCEMENT PROCESS (Figure 14-2)

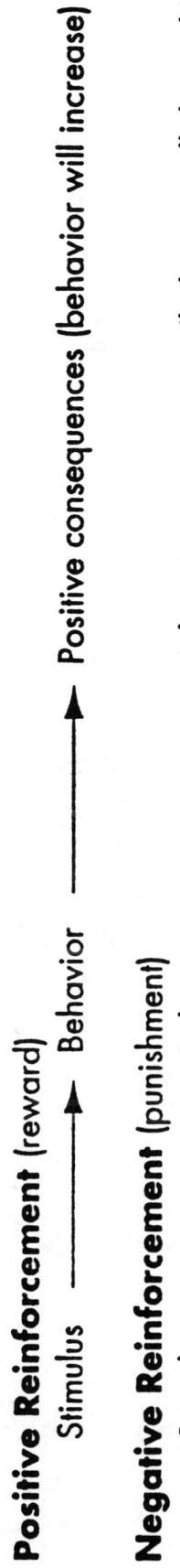

Positive Reinforcement (reward)

Stimulus ———▶ Behavior ———▶ Positive consequences (behavior will increase)

Negative Reinforcement (punishment)

Stimulus ———▶ Behavior ———▶ Adverse consequences (behavior will diminish)

SOCIAL LEARNING THEORY (Figure 14-3)

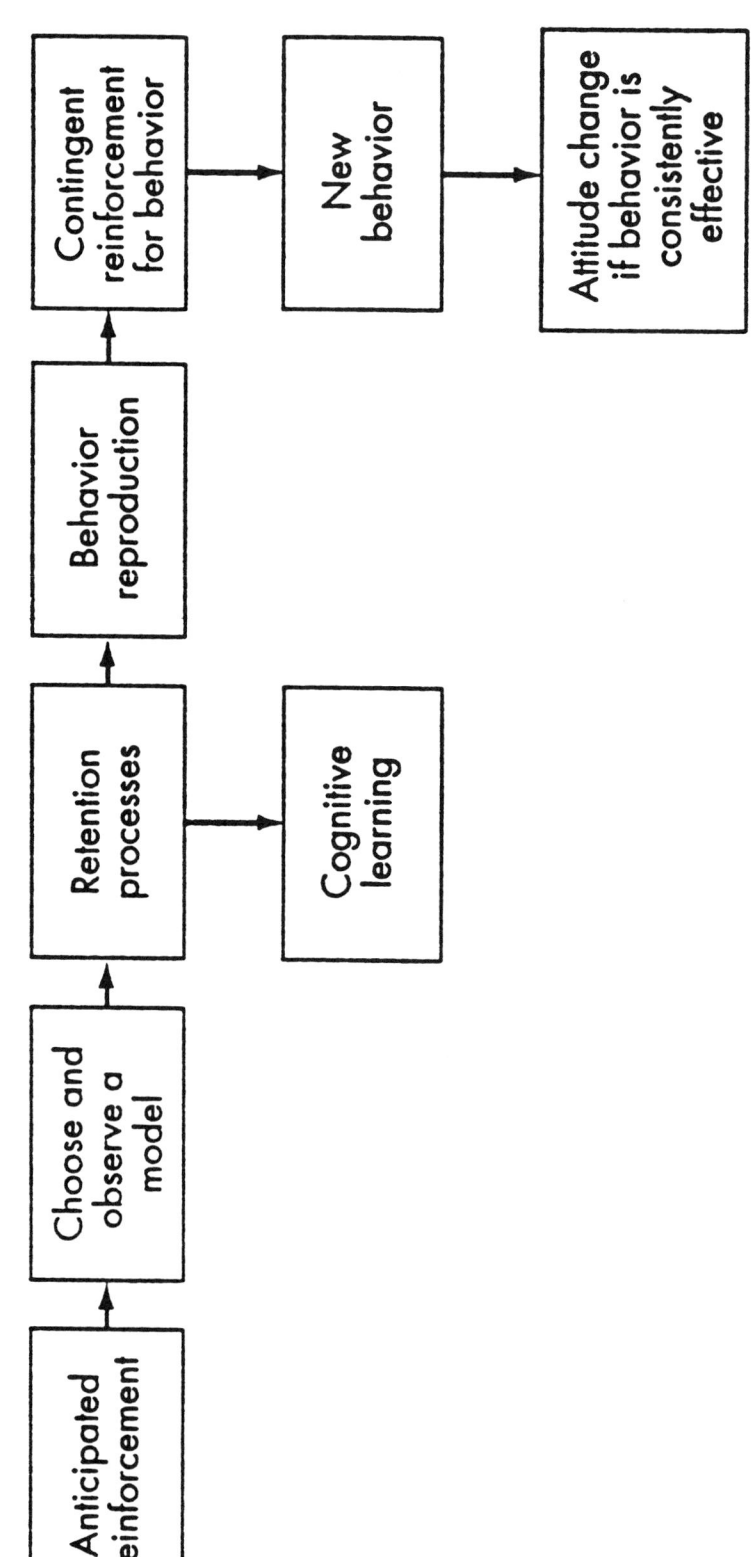

A MODEL OF THE EDUCATIONAL RELAPSE PROCESS (Figure 14-4)

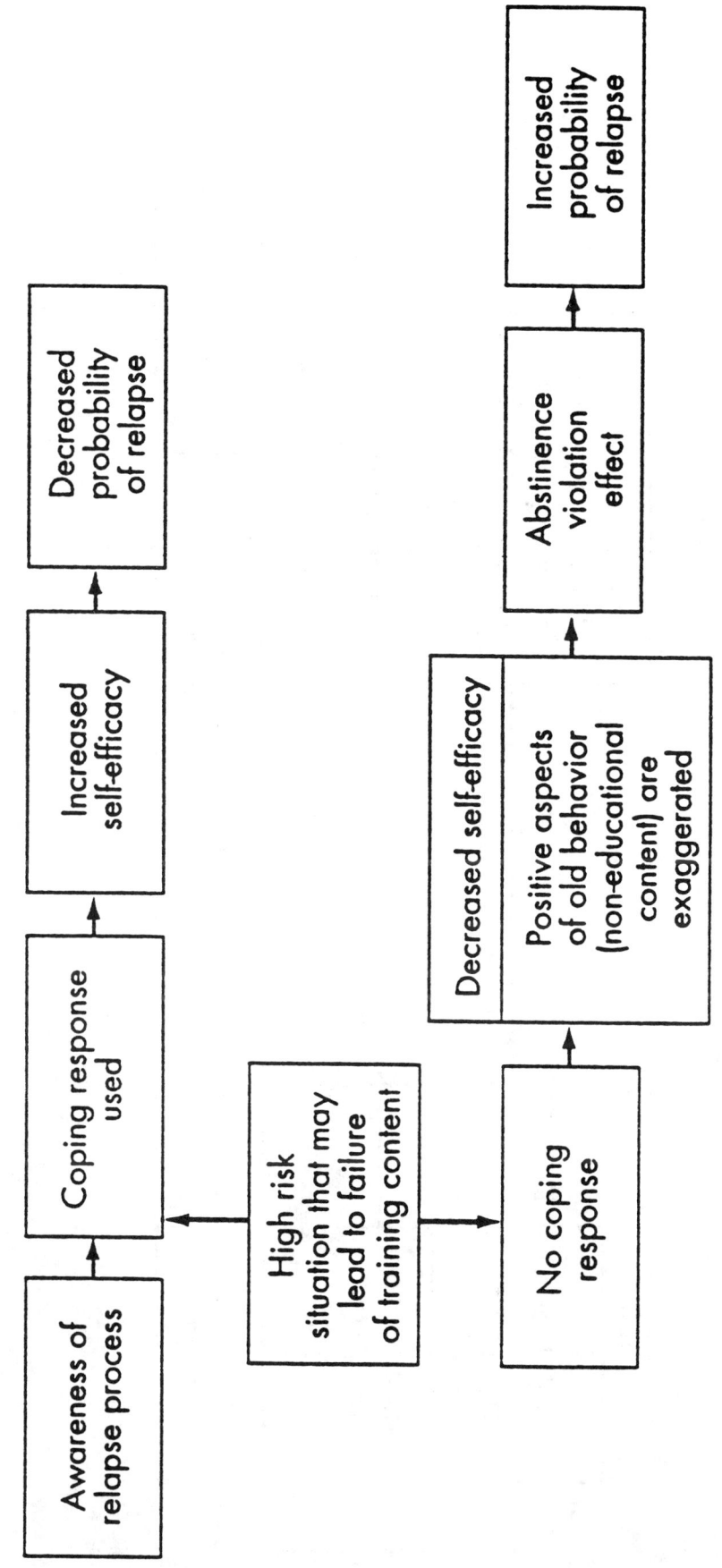

A DIAGNOSTIC MODEL OF EMPLOYEE ATTENDANCE (Figure 17-1)

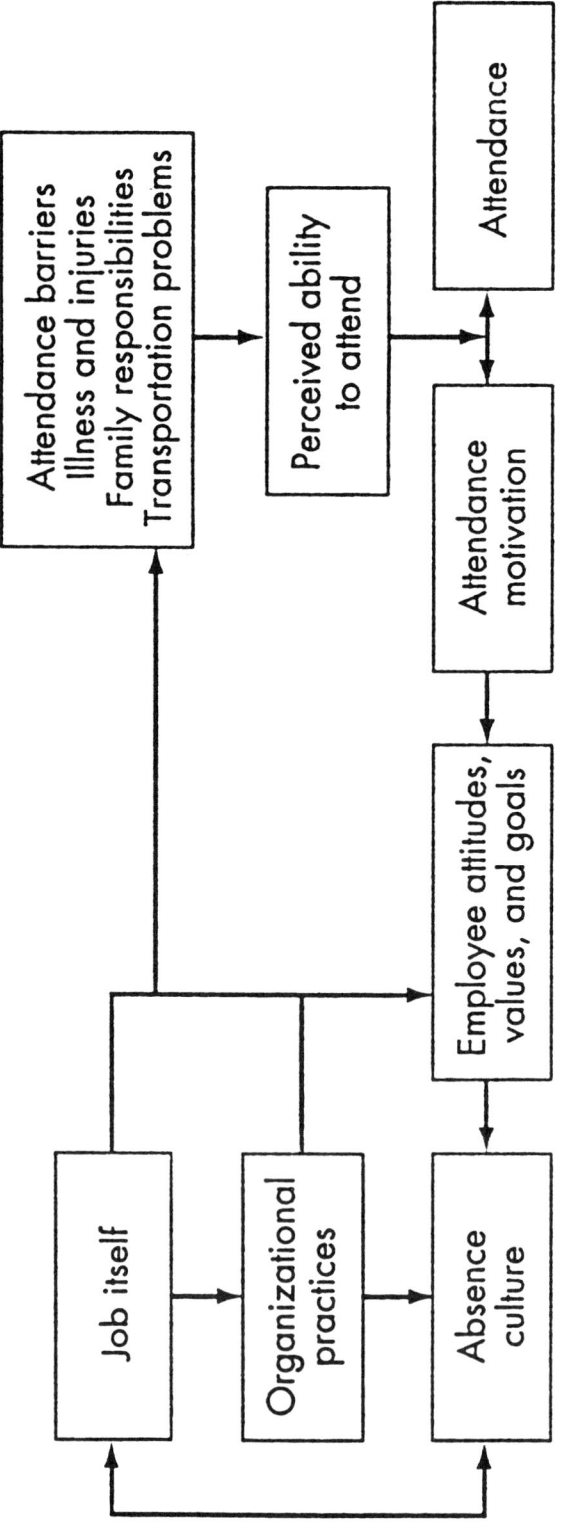

A MODEL OF VOLUNTARY EMPLOYEE TURNOVER (Figure 17-2)

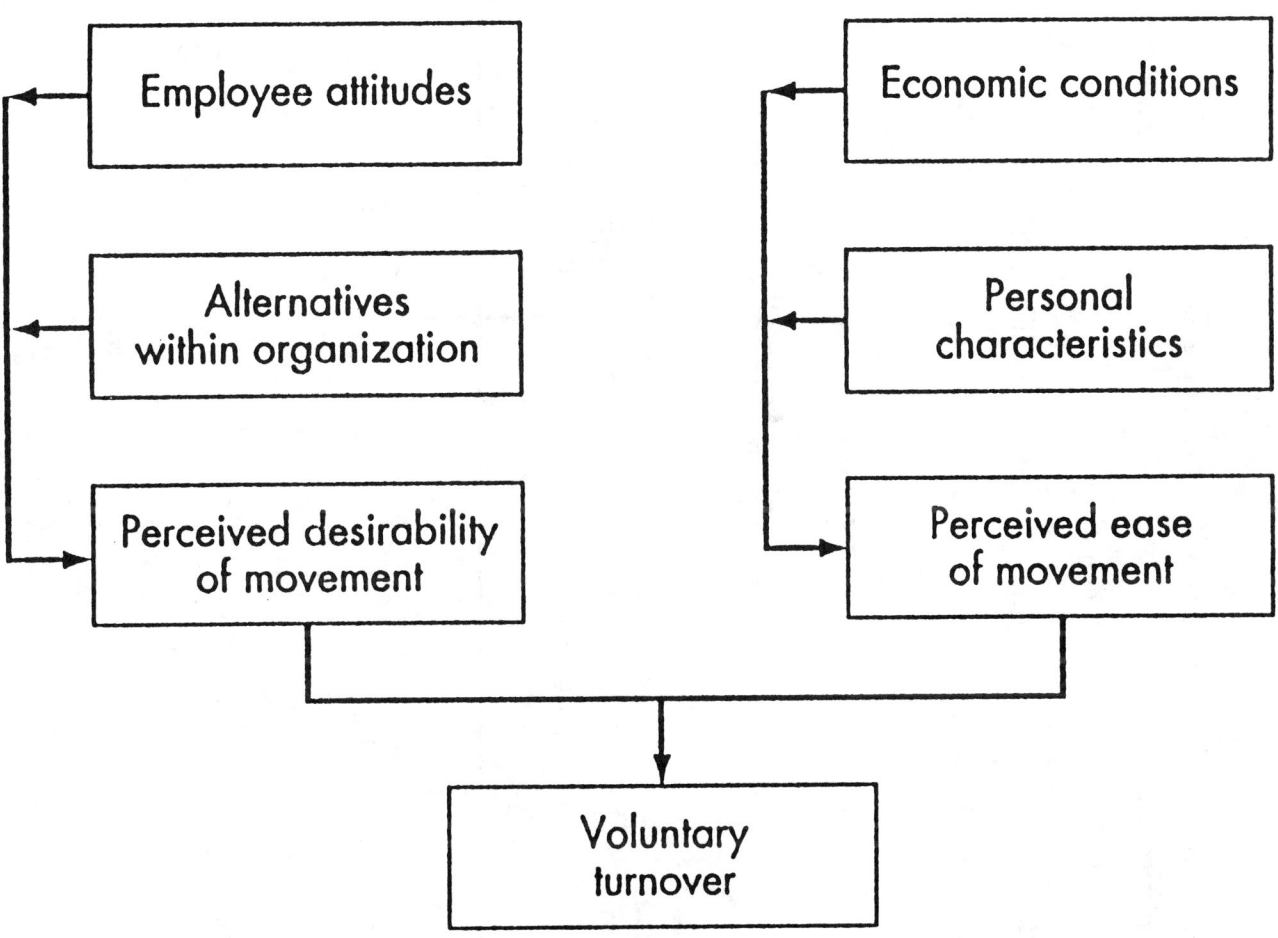

LEWINS'S FORCE-FIELD MODEL OF CHANGE (Figure 20-1)

Restraining forces

Present equilibrium
(status quo)

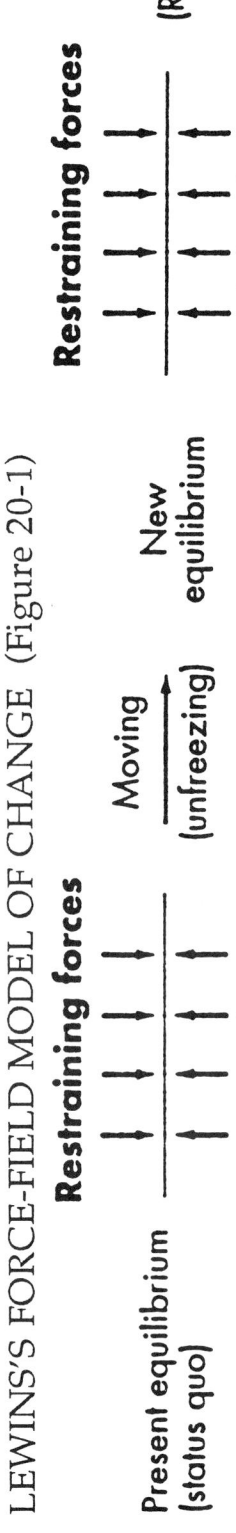

Moving

(unfreezing)

New equilibrium

Driving forces

(Refreezing)

EXAMPLE:

Restraining forces

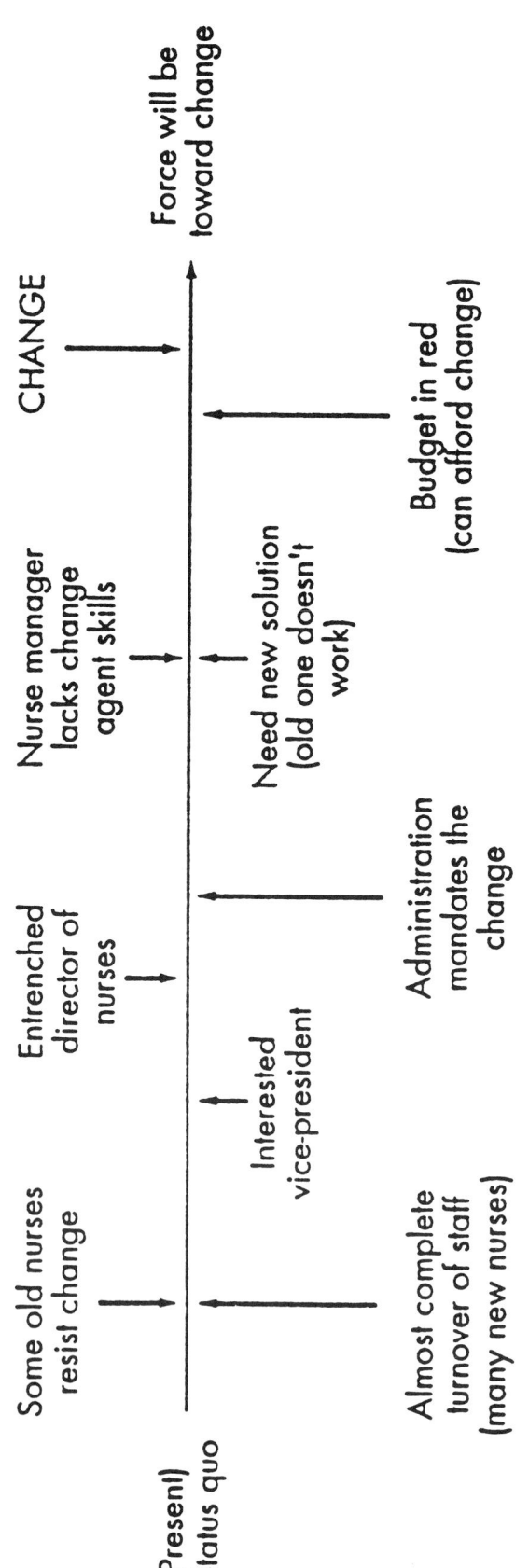

Some old nurses resist change

Entrenched director of nurses

Nurse manager lacks change agent skills

CHANGE

(Present) Status quo

Interested vice-president

Administration mandates the change

Need new solution (old one doesn't work)

Budget in red (can afford change)

Force will be toward change

Driving forces

COMPARISON OF CHANGE MODELS (Figure 20-2)

Lewin	Lippit	Havelock	Rogers
1. Unfreezing	1. Diagnose problem 2. Assess motivation 3. Assess change agent's motivations and resources	1. Building a relationship 2. Diagnosing the problem 3. Acquiring resources	1. Knowledge 2. Persuasion 3. Decision
2. Moving	4. Select progressive change objects 5. Choose change agent role	4. Choosing the solution 5. Gaining acceptance	4. Implementation
3. Refreezing	6. Maintain change 7. Terminate helping relationship	6. Stabilization	5. Confirmation

SEVEN STEPS OF PLANNED CHANGE: AN EXTENSION OF THE
NURSING PROCESS (Figure 20-3)

Nursing Process

Assessment

Planning

Implementation

Evaluation

Change Process

1. Identify the problem or opportunity
2. Collect data
3. Analyze data

4. Plan the change strategies

5. Implement the change

6. Evaluate effectiveness
7. Stablize the change

RISK MANAGEMENT ORGANIZATIONAL MODEL (Figure 21-1)

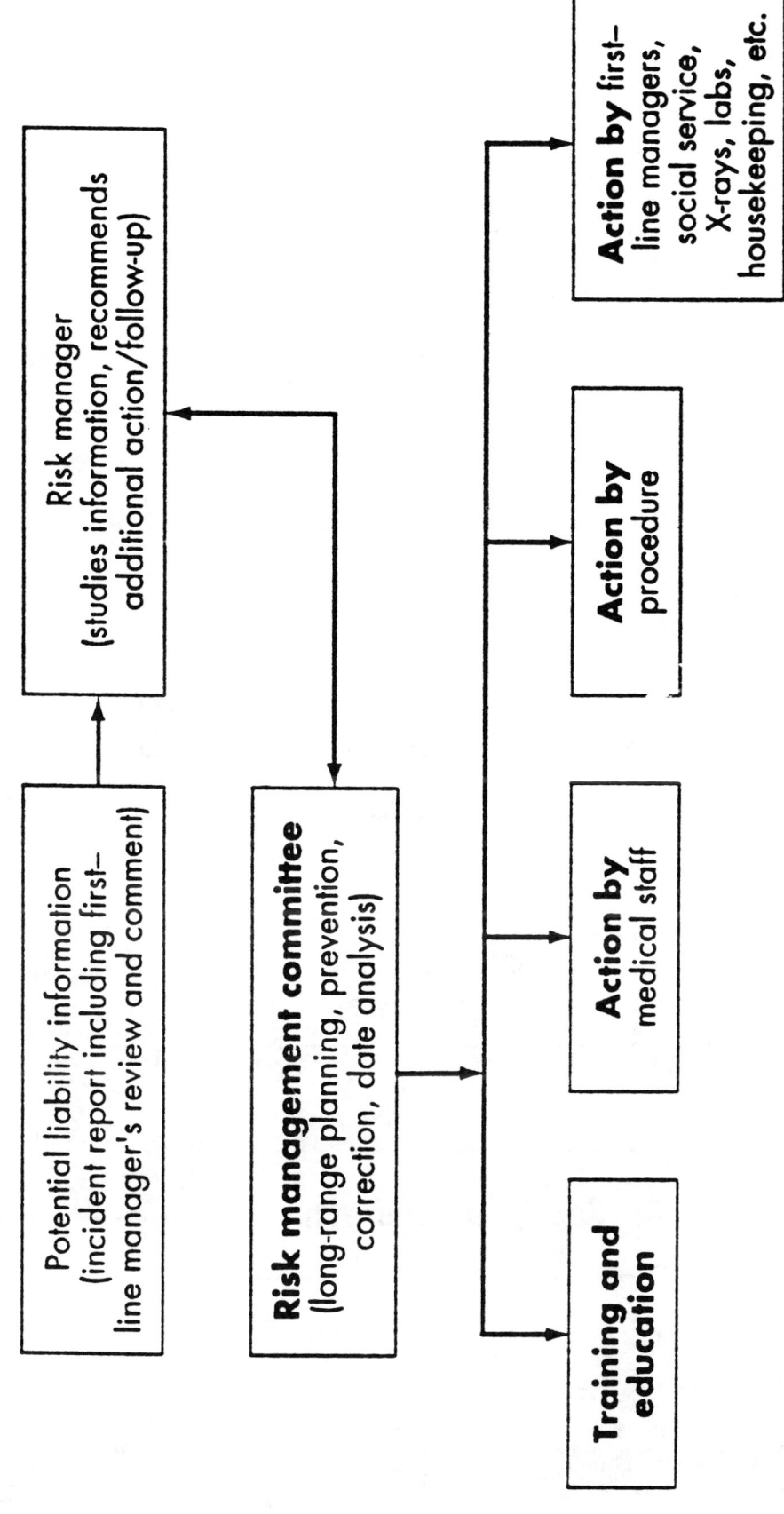

CONFLICT PROCESS (Figure 22-1)

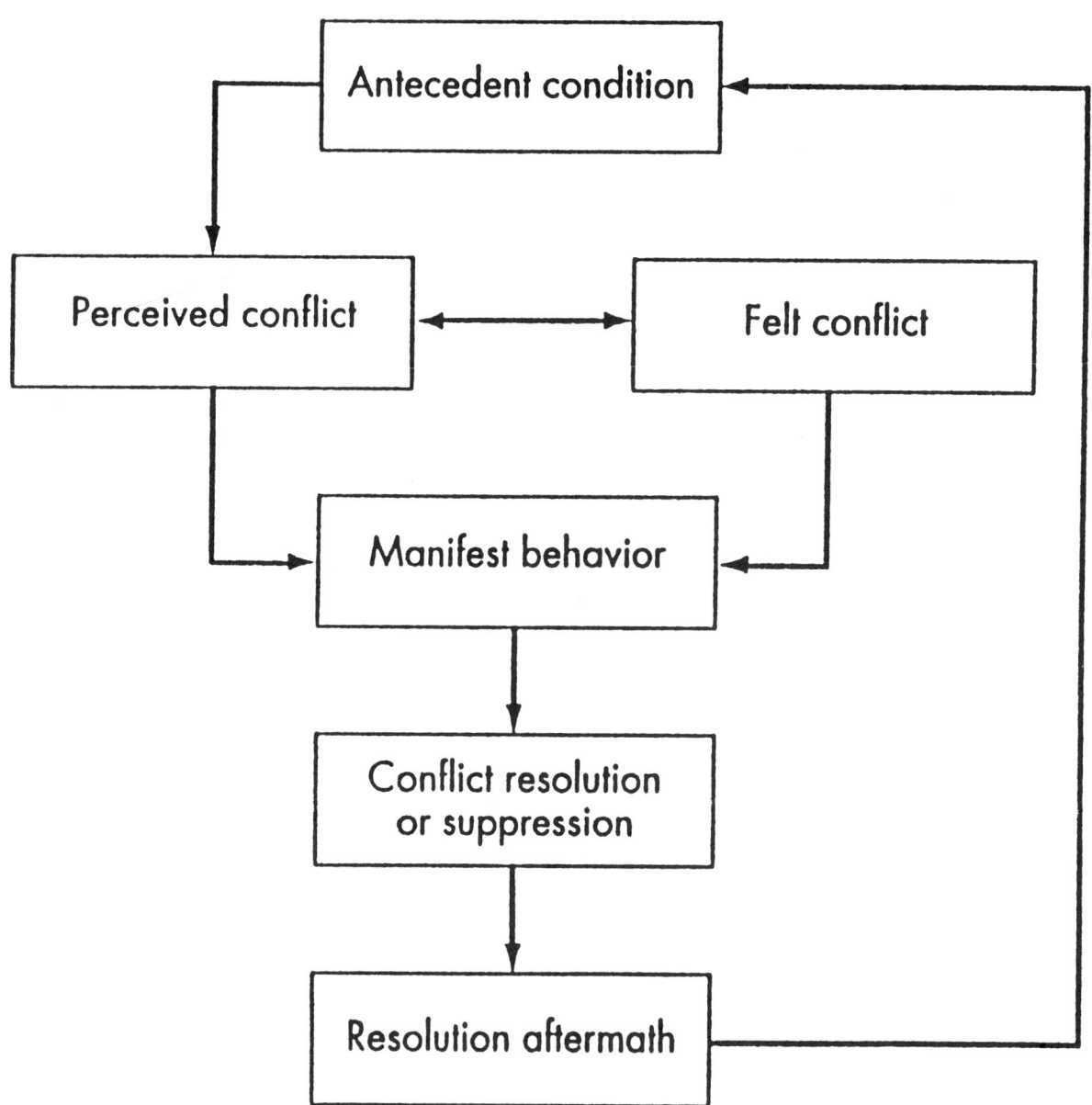